EVERYTHING YOUR OBSTETRICIAN MAY NOT TELL YOU THAT YOU REALLY NEED TO KNOW

You want to do the best for your baby—from the very start. And yet your doctor, no matter how attentive he or she might be, may not take time to tell you all the information contained in this book. The authors, both doctors, have compiled the most accurate facts on all the things you've been wondering about: How does the embryo grow? How should you plan your diet to best serve your baby's needs? What effects do caffeine, nicotine and alcohol have on the fetus, if any? Are the drugs given during labor and delivery safe? What about environmental dangers such as aerosols, paint fumes, X rays, chemicals? These questions, and more are answered fully and clearly in this complete guide to prenatal care.

CARING FOR YOUR UNBORN CHILD

CARING FOR YOUR UNBORN CHILD

BY RONALD E. GOTS, M.D., PH.D. AND BARBARA A. GOTS, M.D.

CARING FOR YOUR UNBORN CHILD

*A Bantam Book | published by arrangement with
Stein and Day, Inc.*

PRINTING HISTORY

*Stein and Day edition published September 1977
2nd printing .. December 1977   3rd printing .... March 1978
Young Parents Books Club edition | January 1978
Serialized in Good Housekeeping | January 1978*

*Bantam edition | August 1979
2nd printing .... February 1980
3rd printing .... March 1981*

ISBN 0-553-20011-9

Published simultaneously in the United States and Canada

Bantam Books are published by Bantam Books, Inc. Its trademark, consisting of the words "Bantam Books" and the portrayal of a bantam, is Registered in U.S. Patent and Trademark Office and in other countries. Marca Registrada. Bantam Books, Inc., 666 Fifth Avenue, New York, New York 10103.

PRINTED IN THE UNITED STATES OF AMERICA

12 11 10 9 8 7 6 5 4 3

To our children, Jason and Meredith,
and to all mothers and their children,
past, present, and future.

CONTENTS

CARING
FOR
YOUR
UNBORN
CHILD

Section One

UNDERSTANDING PREGNANCY

I

The Pregnant Woman Is a New Mother

A three-week-old infant lies propped in her* yellow plastic baby carrier, her right hand clutching a martini. Perhaps there's a cup of coffee grasped in her tiny fingers or a cigarette between her lips. Absurd images? Not really—for the infant is an unborn child, and she may be subjected daily to doses of alcohol, caffeine and nicotine.

After the child is born, her mother is a devoted provider. She tenderly breast-feeds her, if she has been well-advised, and later she carefully plans her infant's menu and selects her food with loving care. All of the rules of good eating hammered home in her home economics classes suddenly come alive. "Balanced diet," an expression filed away in the back of her mind, bursts into consciousness. Now she understands what those teachers meant. In her school days those lessons didn't seem to apply to her, but to someone else. This tiny baby—her newfound responsibility—is that someone else.

Imagine this new mother popping a pill into the mouth of her fretful newborn. Would she ever give her a tranquilizer, an aspirin tablet, a cough remedy or liq-

*Throughout the book the unborn child will either be referred to as "he" or "she." This will circumvent the cumbersome use of "he or she" for each description. We realize that the child may be male or female and will try to give equal time.

uid sleeping medicine from her druggist's display without explicit instructions from her baby's physician? Would she consider for one moment sharing her morning coffee, evening cocktail, or after-breakfast cigarette with this infant. Of course not! She wouldn't dream of exposing her newborn to any potential danger no matter how remote the risk. But she might treat her unborn child, an even more vulnerable creature, in exactly this way.

The growing child is least pampered at a time in her life when she most needs special care: before she is born. As her organs and vital structures grow, she passes through several critical stages. Then, more than ever again, she is particularly vulnerable to attack by drugs, environmental hazards and poor nutrition. Fortunately, there is a great deal the pregnant woman can do to help insure the safe passage of her child through those weeks and months of early growth.

She must start thinking of herself not as a mother-to-be, but as a new mother. Motherhood and mother's responsibility begins from the moment of conception. Her unborn child deserves the same tender love that she lavishes on her newborn. When she eats well, her baby eats well. When she keeps away from unnecessary drugs, reduces her cigarette and coffee consumption and avoids dangers in her environment, her baby benefits from her thoughtfulness. When, on the other hand, she eats a concoction of unbalanced foods, this becomes her baby's diet. The aspirin she takes, the aerosol sprays she breathes, the nicotine, caffeine and artificial sweeteners she consumes are swiftly shuttled into her baby's delicate tissues.

Despite a common misconception, the fetus is not safely sheltered from external assaults. The belief that the mother's womb and placenta magically extract only those good and necessary nutrients the mother has to offer, carefully excluding harmful agents, is absolutely wrong! On the contrary, most of the things mother takes in through her lungs, her digestive tract and her skin are captured by the cells and tissues of the growing baby like a sponge absorbing a puddle of water. They bathe those newly forming cells and become the environment in which they grow.

When they get into the baby's tissues, they may pass through with no ill effects, or they may injure those growing structures. Injuries may be inconsequential like a birth mark on the skin, devastating and fatal like a major organ failure, or somewhere in between in severity. Drugs, viruses, environmental agents, food additives may interfere with the smooth flow of organ development to produce malformations—the so-called "congenital anomalies" or "birth defects." How well we all remember the Thalidomide disaster of the 1960s. This seemingly harmless drug, used to control the annoying symptoms of morning sickness, produced thousands of children with absent or shriveled limbs. German measles, a minor illness for the mother, mercilessly attacks the growing fetus, leaving heart defects, deafness and blindness in its wake.

Thalidomide and German measles are known enemies that can be effectively controlled. Unfortunately, other potential hazards, less dramatic or less predictable in their effects, remain unidentified. But they are important, for congenital malformations are the greatest single killers of children under one year of age. Milder birth defects occur all too frequently—in two percent or more of live births. The incidence is rising and may continue to do so as mothers—and the rest of us—use more and more of the innumerable chemicals that flood our world. Drugs for every ill, artificial sweeteners to remove those few extra pounds, aerosol sprays and household cleaners—an endless list, with new ones added every year.

Fortunately, not all chemicals automatically hurt the growing fetus. At times even potentially harmful chemicals do no damage. They may be inactivated by the cell's protective mechanisms; they may arrive in insufficient quantity to muster a strong attack; they may enter at the wrong time of the growth cycle to cause harm. Many babies come out all right no matter how carelessly their mothers treat them before birth. But why expose the unborn child to avoidable risks? There are many simple steps that you can take that could spell the difference between a normal, healthy child and a severely handicapped one.

Our unborn children have special needs which only their mothers can fulfill. To do that, mothers must first understand the unique problems of the developing child; be aware of the remarkable interrelationship they share, and appreciate the marvelous events of early growth.

This book brings a message of hope to all of you who are pregnant or may be in the future. You can take some simple steps that will help to insure the well-being of your growing child. You can learn how and what to eat, and what "routine" household items—drugs, chemicals and others—that you should temporarily put aside. A new breed of scientist is studying how the food you eat affects your growing child; how the drugs and chemicals that you swallow travel into and alter those maturing tissues; how hair sprays, aerosol deodorants, and other volatile chemicals may be absorbed by the growing fetus. A great deal is still unknown, but many of the answers are in. It's time to share what we know and can infer with those who most need to be informed: you, the new mothers of unborn children.

II

Is It Worth the Risk?

It's that time again: the moment you've been dreading for the past week. The waiting room is packed with young women. The office seems even more crowded and frenetic than usual. Dozens of women, some with figures still trim, others ready to deliver any day, fill the two couches and rows of armchairs.

"Urine specimen please," demands the nurse in a polite, but impersonal manner as she shoves the plastic container into your hand. "As soon as you're done, go into the first room and undress."

In you go, first into the bathroom, then into room number one for the fifth time in as many months.

"No matter how often I go through this I'll never get used to it," you think to yourself as you slip into the drafty open-backed gown.

"Up in the stirrups. The doctor will be with you in a moment," chants the nurse. "Patient ready, Jean?" asks the doctor as he closes the door behind him.

"All set."

"Well, hello, Mrs. Jones. How are you feeling? Any problems since last time?"

"Well, as a matter of fact doctor, . . ."

"You look just fine. Any questions you wanted to ask me?"

You had several questions you wanted to ask. You were concerned because your three-year-old came down with chicken pox last week. You were wondering whether you should cut down on the diet sodas because of

7

that article you read. Maybe if you speak fast you'll be able to get the questions out before he interrupts you again.

"Well, actually, doctor . . ."

Before another word gets out a shock runs through the lower part of your body and stops you cold.

"Just relax. This will just be a little uncomfortable," the doctor says reassuringly as he shoves the speculum far inside.

"Damn! Why do they keep those damn things in the refrigerator?" you ask yourself.

"Did you start to ask something, Mrs. Jones? Was there something you wanted to know?"

There you are, knees in the air, spread far apart, an ice-cold metal gadget in your vagina, with the doctor talking, not to your face, but directly between your legs —almost as if he expected your answer to come from that part of your anatomy.

You think for a moment.

"Oh, what was it I wanted to ask him, anyway?"

You draw a blank. Those questions so carefully rehearsed have vanished.

"How can I possibly have a conversation in this position?" you ask yourself.

"Well, everything looks fine from this end. We'll see you in two weeks."

Out comes the speculum. The door opens and closes.

"You know, I never even saw his face," you think to yourself. "Well, I suppose we're even," you chuckle, trying hard to keep your sense of humor.

Of course, not all obstetricians treat their patients this abruptly. Many can and do take the time to sit and answer questions. Many, acutely aware of the concerns that you have, cheerfully offer advice and reassurance. But even if your obstetrician is a kindly person who makes an effort to chat with you and give you the comfort that you need, he can't possibly answer all of the questions that pop in and out of your mind. First of all, you probably won't remember everything you wanted to ask. Secondly, worries which seem earthshaking to you (as well they should) may be trivial to even the most sympathetic obstetrician—he's heard them a thousand times before.

Perhaps the experience of our friend Mrs. Jones strikes a familiar note, or you may have a warm, considerate obstetrician, but find that you invariably forget most of those nagging questions once inside the doctor's inner sanctum. Do you have countless daily questions which occur to you—too many to call about or to list for your next visit? If so, this book is dedicated to you.

We have tried to explore many of the do's and don't's that bother most pregnant women. We have also added many of our own, taken from the latest medical research.

Our aim is your child's safety. Our goal, to bring the most up-to-date information from the laboratory into your home for you to use. This path from the laboratory to the home has been full of detours and barriers, for there is still so much to learn. Certain aspects of all of our topics, including proper nutrition for the growing baby, hazards in the environment, concerns about the drugs you take, are still in the stages of laboratory research. Many of the messages that we bring are, therefore, preliminary, but they are unquestionably the best and safest recommendations available today.

Purists might object to what may seem to be premature popularization of inconclusive data or to offering you advice which may someday fall by the wayside. We believe this is wrong, for is it reasonable to gamble with the health of your children while we await ironclad proof? "Certainly not!" is our conclusion, and we are sure that most of you will agree. Our intent is not to scare, but to inform. If there is even a shred of evidence that a drug, an everyday household product, a cosmetic might be detrimental to the growing child, you mothers need to know.

We have aimed for the ideal blend of scientific fact and scientific speculation to give you, the pregnant woman, useful, reliable advice. How have we done this? By analyzing every subject and balancing potential risks to your child against possible advantages to you or your child. When a potential risk is small or uncertain, we tell you so. We do not make dogmatic recommendations from scanty data. We do offer the facts as they now exist and give you the opportunity to make your own choice.

When you are pregnant, you take chances for two people. What's more, the other person may be far more vulnerable to certain risks than you are. Whatever you eat, inhale or rub on your skin should be sufficiently important to you to justify the risk, however small, to your unborn child. Potential dangers, highly speculative or unproven, are remote risks. If they are a necessary part of your life, they may well be worth the small chance you take. If they are frills, you may want to put them aside during your pregnancy. This concept—risk versus benefit—is repeated time and again throughout this book. You must understand this principle completely before going any further.

Certain undertakings may be so integrated into our lives that we never consciously weigh the advantages against the disadvantages. Other activities, unfamiliar to us or a bit scary, may make us pause and ponder.

"Should we take the chance? Is it worth it?"

For example, the empty cupboard shouts its familiar reminder. "Time to go to the supermarket again."

You grab the kids, hop in the car, start the motor and you're off. Do you stop and think, "Hey! We might have an accident and all be killed!" Probably not, for you have no choice. You have to buy the food. The benefit far outweighs the risk, making the choice inescapable.

Every move you make is in some way, subtly or overtly, consciously or subconsciously, guided by the principle of risk versus benefit. If the benefit is great and the risk small—like going to the store—the decision is easy. You go. If the risk is high and the benefit small —like skydiving—the decision for most of you is simple: you don't jump out of the plane.

Between these extremes are many personal and individual choices that only you can make. They depend on your personal needs, desires, lifestyles and concerns. Occasionally we have taken the liberty here of giving our assessment of benefit. We do this for those hazards which seem to be unessential frills of modern society and which, we feel, most women can live comfortably without. In most cases, however, we simply present the facts and leave the choice to you. Throughout we have tried to view these matters through the eyes of the pregnant woman.

We ask, "Would you use a roll-on, cream or pad deodorant, if there were even the slightest chance that the aerosol types might harm your child?"

"Of course!" you would probably answer. "I can certainly change deodorants for those nine months. But I had no idea. . . ."

Would you refrain from painting a poorly ventilated room if we told you that the volatile chemicals that fill your nose and lungs might damage his growing tissues?

"Certainly!" you would likely reply. "What good is a cheerful bright room, if he can't enjoy it? Anyway, this provides an excuse to make my husband do the painting."

Would you do without the diet drinks, if there were even the slightest possibility that those artificial sweeteners could be harmful?

For most of you the answer would be simple and unhesitating:

"I'll switch back to the sugar-containing ones. That won't upset me a bit."

Ah, but would you give up smoking?

To that question you ponder longer. "Is it really dangerous? I smoked before and all of my other children are okay. Many of my friends smoke, and their children are normal."

You must make your own decision. The risk to your unborn child is small but well proven. The benefit is something only you can assess.

Would you get rid of your cat, if you knew that his presence threatened your child's eyesight?

"But I really love my cat," you reply.

We understand that, but will caution you quite strongly at least to have someone else empty the litter box. That will improve your child's safety immeasurably.

We hope we haven't been too presumptuous in answering some of these questions for you. We suspect that most of you will agree with many of our answers. If not, you will make your own choices, but with your eyes open, knowing the available facts.

We ask and attempt to answer other queries dealing with nutrition, food additives, drugs and environmental exposures. Here are some of them.

- Are the drugs the doctor gives me for morning sickness really safe?
- What can I do if I get a cold or a headache? Can I take aspirin or cold remedies?
- Can my smoking cigarettes or drinking alcoholic beverages affect my child?
- What foods should I eat and which should I avoid? Should I take vitamin and iron supplements?
- How much weight can I safely gain? My doctor tells me to keep my weight down. Is this correct?
- What if I need an operation while I am pregnant? Is this safe for the baby?
- What if I have a serious condition like diabetes, epilepsy or high blood pressure? Can I take my medications without worry?
- What do cats and rare meat have in common? Can they really affect my baby's eyesight?
- Can I spray my house or garden with insecticides, fungicides or fertilizers while I am pregnant?
- Might the hair dyes that I use damage my baby?
- What about artificial sweeteners? Are they safe?
- Am I working at a job that exposes my unborn child to unusual hazard?

Many of the answers will probably surprise you.

This is not a fire-and-brimstone scare book. Nothing could be worse for the growing child than a nail-biting, anxiety-laden mother frantic about things that she cannot control or overly worried about uncertain hazards.

Instead, it is a book of hope. We offer easy-to-follow recommendations that will not turn your life upside down. We believe that you modern women are unwilling to play ostrich, burying your heads in the sand and accepting a philosophy of, "What I don't know can't hurt me (or my child)."

Our intent is to bring forth new insights: first, that you, the pregnant woman, share your world with another person—one who is more vulnerable to assaults than you; second, that there are simple steps that you can take to help your child along.

We will begin our journey into the special and sensitive world of the growing fetus. First, we will follow his growth step-by-step from the moment of conception to the day he leaves his mother's womb. Let us live through his development and learn what easy things his mother can do to influence his progress most favorably toward normal growth and good health.

III

The Baby Grows

One hundred million sperm cells propelled by their thrashing tails swim upstream toward a single egg or ovum. When they arrive, only one, perhaps stronger or faster than the rest, can fight its way inside. The sperm and ovum merge, become a single unit and set into motion a remarkable chain of events. From that moment on the mysterious process of reproduction marches forward with a predictable rhythm and an astounding accuracy. Time and time again a new human being is created, flawless in form and structurally identical to millions before him. But occasionally the cadence is broken and the process goes awry. Mistakes occur which mar this usually precise flow of human reproduction.

These mistakes take many forms: organs may be misshapen or absent; harmful or fatal chemical imbalances may occur; miscarriages may interrupt the pregnancy; the infant may be born prematurely before he is fully prepared to face the world; the vulnerable newborn may be threatened by impaired resistance or by harmful drugs carried from his mother's blood into his system at that critical moment just before birth.

Some of these mishaps are beyond the mother's control. Certain genetic mismatches or mysterious events are unavoidable. But many threats to the growing fetus can be eliminated or reduced. You can help insure the safe development of your growing child, if you only know how.

14

The developing fetus teeters on a narrow precipice, delicately balanced between smooth and proper formation and potential failure or error. His programmed, orderly maturation is exquisitely timed and fine tuned. Any interruption of this natural rhythm will disrupt the necessary sequence and may throw off all of the subsequent steps. This rhythmic growth process is controlled by inherited genetic information, but it is fueled and modified by influences from outside.

The child's contact with the outside world comes through the placenta via his mother's womb. The placenta is a living sponge which soaks up nutrients from the mother's blood and passes them to the growing child. It carries the life-building substances that form the tissues of this new individual. It can also carry chemical toxins and microorganisms which are harmless to the mature tissues of the mother but a menace to newly forming organs. Thus the child's environment is intimately related to its mother's. To appreciate this closest-of-all relationships and to sense the unusual susceptibility of fetal tissues to assaults from outside, we must follow the process of fetal growth from conception to birth.

Human development is so complex that it boggles the imaginations of most of us. No one understands it completely, but scientists have worked out many of the precise, interconnected steps. It is far beyond the scope of this book to cover all of those details or to try to turn you into embryologists (students of fetal development). Those of you who want a more detailed picture may refer to any of the references listed in the bibliography section. For our present purposes you need enough general understanding of the steps that precede the birth of your child to appreciate your role: to see how the foods you eat, the drugs you take, the things you breathe might affect your child. We will therefore embark together on a very simplified journey through those nine months before birth when your baby lives within you. We will concentrate on those periods of greatest danger when he most needs your help.

Conception

Life begins in the fallopian tube, the four-inch passageway that connects the ovary to the uterus. The ovary releases the ovum or egg into the fallopian tube. This is called ovulation. The sperm must fertilize that ovum within one to three days after ovulation, before it passes through the fallopian tube and into the uterus. Millions of sperm from the male, minute compared with the relatively massive ovum (see figure 1 for actual size of ovum), must compete. After a sperm gets inside, the membrane of the ovum staunchly repels any other intruders.

The ovum and sperm are special reproductive cells, different from all other cells of the body. Every other cell—e.g., cells of the muscles, white blood cells, fat cells, brain cells—have 46 sets of chromosomes, the information centers contained within each cell nucleus that controls all cellular functions. In a very real sense the chromosomes are the computers of the cells. They are also the storehouses of information passed from generation to generation. They make us like our grandfathers, but different from our neighbors' grandfathers. They determine the color of our hair, our eyes and our skin. They set the pattern for the shapes of our eyes, our ears and our noses. They tell our bodies how tall they can grow and, to some extent, how long they can live. The sperm and ovum differ from all other cells in that they contain only half the number of chromosomes. Instead of 46, they have 23. This permits them to unite and to form a new complete cell carrying 46 chromosomes, half of which come from the mother, half from the father. That is exactly what happens as soon as the sperm enters the ovum. Within moments their chromosomes meld together to form a new complete single cell—the control center for a new individual.

For the next two to three days this cell is a busy creature, engaged simultaneously in two separate activities. It divides over and over again to form a grape-like mass of daughter cells, identical to itself, and it journeys down the fallopian tube toward the uterus where it will reside for the next nine months. By the end of those two to three active days, the incipient individual is composed of approximately 32 cells and it now has a name of its very own—the morula (figure 1).

Shortly after the morula enters its mother's uterus, it bursts into a new and different flurry of activity. The marvelous process of differentiation has begun. Differentiation causes cells which were identical to one another to change and take on separate and unique identities. It teaches them what they must do to form specialized tissues and organs which carry out their own peculiar functions.

Just as society depends on each individual—the teacher, the custodian, the doctor, the lawyer—to contribute his special talents for the good of all, so, too, do the different tissues and organs of the body carry out their special activities to serve the whole person. Without differentiation there could be no reproduction and no new person. It commands each cell to behave in its own unique and vital way. It tells the brain cells how to think, the heart muscle cells how to squeeze and pump the blood, the intestinal lining cells how to digest and absorb foods. What's more, it tells the cells when and how to begin coming together to form the kidneys, heart, brain, spinal cord, lungs, stomach and other organs. Equally remarkable, it tells them when to stop, for it knows when the job is done and the organ is fully formed.

Another amazing thing about differentiation is that every cell in the body contains the same chromosomes. They all have the identical computer program with 46 identical chromosomes (except, as we have seen, for the sperm and ovum, which have 23). Yet, they are able to take on their own identities and to form different organs with unique capabilities and characteristics. How do cells manage this? By tuning in, as they differentiate, to only certain bits of genetic information —those messages directed specifically for them. Those differentiating cells act like miniature radios, all capable of receiving all stations, but tuning in to

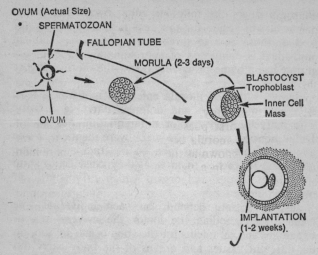

Figure 1 Fertilization and Implantation

only one. Each cell, then, accepts commands from the right genes. Nerve cells listen to signals meant for them, but tune out or turn off signals designed for liver cells. Muscle cells, although theoretically capable of becoming bones, eyes, or lungs, don't. They leave those tasks to other cells. Differentiation is one of nature's great miracles. It starts with identical computer programs, opens some pathways and short-circuits others and ends up with a completed unit of different parts all interacting and cooperating for the good of the whole person.

As you might imagine, differentiation is a most delicate process, susceptible to many chemical and environmental setbacks. If it is in any way interrupted or diverted, the fledgling organism may die before birth or fall victim to a variety of deformities or organ malformations.

Notice that differentiation begins very early in reproduction—only one week after fertilization of the egg by the sperm. This is well before the mother even knows that she is pregnant, for she won't miss her period for another week. Thus, a critical and rapidly changing time in the life of this new baby is well under way before the mother is aware that her offspring is there. Why is this so important? It means that a mother's responsibility begins, not when the doctor gives her the happy news, but before she has any idea she is pregnant. It begins from that moment when she contemplates becoming a new mother, or exposes herself to that possibility.

During the first phases of differentiation, some of the cells of the morula begin to separate and to form an outer layer known as the trophoblast. Others remain centrally located in a tight bundle. This ball-like blob of cells is known as the inner cell mass. Fluid is secreted by some of the cells and accumulates around this central cell mass. Now the tiny growing organism is the size of a pinhead. It looks like a minute blister with an outer and an inner layer of cells and a drop of liquid inside. This small spherical creature is no longer called a morula. It has graduated to a new stage and has proudly changed its name to blastocyst (figure 1).

Implantation

It is the job of the blastocyst to find a comfortable home in the inner recesses of the mother's uterus. Approximately one week after the sperm fought its way inside the ovum, this blastocyst burrows its way into the lining of the womb. In a sense it is like a living animal which digs and tunnels until it finds safe refuge underground. Instead of digging, the blastocyst depends upon various chemical substances that it secretes. These dissolve the mother's tissues, opening a pathway into which it can cozily nestle. The uterine lining assists in this task, for at this stage, after fertilization, the mother's hormones have given it a spongy, pliable consistency—an inviting host for this new guest (figure 1).

Probably half of all pregnancies fail at this stage of implantation. For any one of hundreds of reasons, many of which are still mysteries of nature, the womb rejects this intruder. When it does, a normal menstrual period follows shortly thereafter, and the woman never knows that she was a potential mother.

Weeks Two and Three

The next two weeks find this creature busy day and night in an endless flurry of activity. One would think that he would get tired and need to rest, but he never does. His cells divide and redivide. Differentiation becomes more widespread until the basic patterns for all of the different organs are laid down. Parts of the tiny embryo are designated as food gatherers. They burrow deeper into the uterine lining, sending out rootlike structures called villi which will ultimately form part of the placental unit which brings nutrients from the mother to the tissues of her growing child.

During the second week all of the preliminary stages of differentiation have started. The cells that will form each of the organ systems—the nervous system, the digestive system, the circulatory system, the lungs, skin, muscles, bones and endocrine organs—have begun to separate and to assume individual identities. So have the cells that will help support the baby in its new environment. These include those cells that will make the villi and other parts of the placenta and those that will form the amniotic sac—the balloon-like membrane filled with fluid that covers and protects the growing child in a soft liquid cushion. Before long this growing child will be floating, seemingly weightless, in a watery cocoon.

By the end of the third week the new embryo (some scientists call it a preembryo until it reaches the fourth week) has elongated in shape and has a large sphere known as the yolk sac attached to it. This will be the center of blood formation for the new baby until its mature blood-forming organs—the bone marrow and spleen—are sufficiently grown to take over. The embryo is now surrounded by a thin primitive balloon or amnion. The villi are pressing forward more vigorously every day to tap into and soak up nutrients from the mother's womb. By the end of the third week the embryo is approximately ⅛ inch long, has elongated

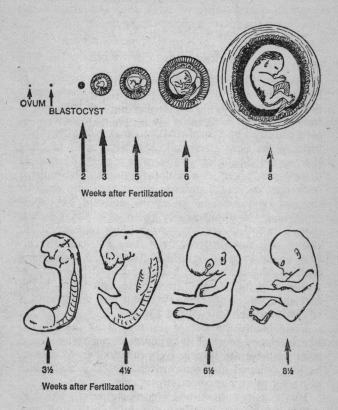

Figure 2 Growth of the embryo and
fetus. Drawings above are about ½ actual size.
Below are not to scale, but show when and
how forms change during development

into a C-like configuration, and is safely surrounded by those cells that will become its protective cover. The entire unit—embryo, yolk sac, and amnion envelope—is the size of a large pea (figure 2).

Weeks Four and Five

By the beginning of the fourth week, this baby is universally called an embryo. The tiny C-shaped mass now calls into play all of those cells that have begun to differentiate. Their jobs are to multiply, grow, fold, turn and twist into forms that will make the vital structures of the new individual. The remarkable molding that occurs during these two weeks make it seem as if they were spent in a sculptor's studio. The embryo undergoes radical changes in shape and form and, by the end of week four, bears the outward basic patterns that are unmistakably those of a living being, though not yet clearly human. How remarkable to realize that this progress from the single-celled fertilized ovum to a recognizable living form containing millions of cells, each with its specialized function, required only four weeks. Even more astonishing is the fact that this new being with all its complexity is still only ¼ inch long (figure 2).

Long before the end of the fifth week the embryo has developed most of its primitive organ systems, and some of these are now actively functioning. Moreover, he has assumed new outward changes that make him distinctly more human in appearance.

His heart is formed and vigorously pumps blood at a rate of 60 to 70 times per minute through tiny blood vessels that are invisible to the naked eye. Kidneys, no larger than a speck of dust, are now present and will soon begin primitive filtering and excretory functions. Certain of the endocrine glands, including the thyroid and adrenals, have taken shape. The central nervous system, consisting of brain and spinal cord, are now laid out in their fundamental forms with all of their separate parts well defined and on their way to full development. Primitive lungs dot the forming chest cavity. They won't be used for many months—

until the newborn child reaches the outside air—but soon there will be some early gasps, some weak and ineffective attempts at breathing in this liquid cocoon where the child resides. The liver, stomach and remainder of the digestive tract have taken their places with the other organs in the inner recesses of this tiny embryo.

External forms, too, are taking shape. By the end of the fourth week primitive limb buds have appeared on the outside of the growing embryo. The almost staggering rapidity of this early growth period is exemplified by that first sprouting of arms and legs. In a 48-hour period the embryo is visibly transformed from a smooth, limbless creature into the bearer of budlike projections. Only a week and a half later, those tiny stumps will have grown and be dotted at the ends by five tiny fingers and toes (figure 2).

The tremendous activity, the differentiation of parts into their special functions, and the division and multiplication of embryonic size is a marvel of nature. Never again in the remaining 70 years of this child's life will his body be in such a state of frenzied activity. Although he is still only ½ inch long at the end of week five, already he has increased in size almost 10,-000 fold since the start of his one-celled life. His total cells have increased by millions, and those cells have advanced from single unspecialized units into a phase of frenetic change and specialization. Every organ and structure that will carry this new individual through his entire life is now well on its way to full development.

It is easy to conceive that this is a time of delicate balance, vulnerability and potential failure. Unlike adult tissues which multiply and reform much more slowly, embryonic tissues expand at a tremendous pace. They need constant support from proper foods to provide the energy and building blocks for this rapid growth. They need constant sheltering from unwanted hazards. They must move forward with uninterrupted precision in order to form normal structures. Any noxious exposures transmitted through the mother's tissues can readily halt or divert this normally smooth, programmed process. The growing embryo, at the mercy of its mother's internal environment, needs pampering and loving protection.

Weeks Six Through Eight

The next three weeks witness further refinements of internal organs and external body structure, and the formation of specialized sensory organs—the eyes, ears and nose. Other organs, less important for life support, but part of the final form of the new being. take shape. Such tissues as muscles, bones, cartilage and skin rapidly develop, endowing this embryo with a progressively more and more human quality (figure 2).

Over these three weeks the eye's lens, cornea and retina, all essential for normal vision, are molded into mature form. Other sensory structures, including those required for hearing and balance, grow concomitantly. Thus weeks six through eight are crucial to the genesis of special sensory functions. Infections or chemical attacks occurring then can lead to the devastating birth defects of blindness and deafness.

Primitive sex organs also form during the latter half of the second month. By the end of week eight, male and female sexual characteristics are recognizable. Certain hazards in the fetal environment during this period can adversely influence normal sexual differentiation.

By the end of the second month the growing organism is no longer known as an embryo, but is now a fetus. Why the distinction? Because now the growing child has all of the basic organ structures needed to sustain him for the remainder of his life. To be sure, there are still a great many fine touches and details remaining to be filled in, but the fundamental framework is there.

All of this astounding activity fled by in two short months. The mother has missed only two periods. She is just beginning to believe that she is really pregnant. Even more striking, the fetus, with all of its complexity, is still only one inch long and weighs less than an ounce. It has arms, legs, ear holes and a primitive face (although its eyelids haven't fully formed and its features are still rather grotesque) and has taken on the appearance of a human creature.

The Third Month

The third month brings further refinement, some new growth and heightened physical activity. The bone marrow begins to specialize into its blood-forming function and replaces the yolk sac as the source of red blood cells which carry oxygen to the baby's tissues. The face becomes even more human as the ears form and the mouth becomes better defined. The eyelids, just developing, are tightly closed and will remain sealed for three more months. The separate parts of the oral cavity come together and fuse, making sucking and swallowing possible. If this fusion goes astray, one of the most common of all birth defects—cleft palate—will be the result.

Soon the fetus begins swallowing some of the amnionic fluid that surrounds him. He will even inhale some of this liquid into his primitive lungs. If we did this we would drown, but it is harmless before birth since the oxygen he needs to support his growth and survival comes not through the lungs, as it does for us, but through the mother's blood. During this third month the fetal kidneys begin to excrete urine into the amnionic fluid—a life-supporting process which accelerates inexorably from that time on: a fact which all new mothers will surely corroborate.

As new structural tissues are laid down, the baby's bones and muscles strengthen. He now moves around actively, exercising those muscles, feeling his new world, and using the pathways from his newly functioning nervous system that tell his muscles how to move. In a sense, the baby is beginning to learn, and movement is the first phase of his education. The fetus still is too small for the mother to detect any of these movements. By the end of three months he is only two to three inches long.

The Fourth Month

By now all that remains are some finishing touches and further growth in size and strength before the child is ready to take his place beside, rather than inside, his mother.

Now the baby receives its nourishment through the placenta. He pumps his blood not just round and round his own body as he did before, but through the umbilical arteries that lead to the placenta and back through the umbilical vein, returning the blood, now oxygenated, to his own circulation. His heart is strong and it pumps the blood at a rapid and vigorous rate.

The story of placental circulation and of the placenta itself is the backbone of this book, for it describes the relationship between the fetus, its mother and the outside world. All foods necessary for growth and all chemicals potentially harmful find their way into the baby by this route. This relationship between baby, mother and the world outside will be discussed in great detail as we delve deeper into the world of the fetal environment.

During the fourth month fine features of the face and body become more babylike. The fetus grows fine hair covering most of its skin, and tiny fingernails now make their appearance.

This month brings rapid growth in both length and weight. The baby increases in size from the 3 to 4 inches of the previous month to a length of 8 to 10 inches, nearly half as long as he will be at birth. As he grows, he lays down more structural tissues. His muscles become stronger, his body more solid. Now the mother begins to appreciate his existence, for during this month the first early flutters of kicks and turns formally announce the presence of this new individual. Now, too, the doctor can unequivocally tell that a living baby is growing inside, for he can hear the heart beat by using a special sensitive stethoscope. If there are twins, he will soon be able to give the mother the good (or bad) news, for two separate heartbeats will come through loud and clear.

The Fifth and Sixth Months

Except for its diminutive size, the baby is nearly fully formed by the end of the fifth month. This is the halfway point in his intrauterine development, for in 20 more weeks he will be born. By now he is 12 inches long and weighs over a pound. Because he is still very small and his lungs and brain are immature, he cannot survive if he is removed from the protective environment within his mother. He is not quite self-sufficient.

Twenty weeks or five months marks the last time when the normal pregnancy can legally be terminated by abortion. After this time the fetus rapidly approaches the point when he can survive on his own. Moreover, after 20 weeks the increasing size of the fetus makes most abortion techniques unduly risky for the mother. Whether the fetus is a living individual by now is a matter of philosophical and theological debate. It is also a current raging social argument. The answer depends entirely upon one's philosophy. The fetus does have many inner and outward characteristics of a human being, but at 20 weeks he is not an independent living creature.

For the remainder of these two months the baby adds more bulk, length and physical strength. He gets more body hair, and his nails begin to grow long. Eyebrows and eyelashes make their first appearances. His body elongates and the trunk and legs lengthen rapidly, increasing in proportion to the head which earlier comprised the majority of the fetal length.

By the sixth month the baby is probably aware of his environment. His small brain is beginning to wonder about the things around him. His eyelids are now fully formed, and he has muscular control over them. Quite likely he opens and closes his eyes. He may even be able to see some faint light diffused through the mother's abdominal wall. He stretches his arms and legs, exercising his new muscles and testing the control of his nervous system. He may even suck his thumb as he explores his world and body. His auditory senses are well developed, and he hears and can respond to sounds from the outside. He may be startled, as most mothers know, and respond with kicks and pushes when disturbed by a slamming door or a falling pot.

Now he begins to put heavier demands on his mother, for he requires all of the nourishment that she can provide to support this burgeoning growth. By the end of the sixth month the child weighs approximately two pounds. If he is born now he will probably die, since his lungs and brain are still quite immature, but with the best modern hospital care he might make it. A number of babies weighing two pounds or less have survived and grown into healthy, normal adults.

The Last Three Months

There are a few final touches in organ maturation, particularly in the lungs and brain, which occur during the final three months. However, this is mostly a period of growth rather than fine adjustment. The baby increases rapidly in size, making even greater demands on his mother's reserves. He begins to accumulate heavy layers of fat under his skin which make him soft and cuddly and will pad and insulate his body and supply some of his early nutritional needs after he emerges from his mother.

Environmental, chemical, viral and drug hazards rarely lead to significant organ defects from this point on, since the organs are for the most part fully formed. If the baby has come through the first six months normally developed, he will be born without any organ malformations. But he isn't completely out of the woods, for his bodily defenses are still weak and he can still fall victim to other hazards. Instead of producing organ malformations, certain hazards during these last three months may cause organs to fail, chemical imbalances to occur, or units such as the brain to function improperly. They may even kill the still vulnerable fetus before birth or shortly after delivery. Thus, the last three months are still critical and precarious times. The expectant mother must never relax her attentive nurturing.

Now, with every passing week, the child's chances

for independent survival increase. Every day, week, month he becomes larger, stronger and better able to face the world on his own. By the time he weighs three and a half pounds, at the end of seven months, his chances of surviving, given optimal care, are fair. Once he has reached five pounds, approximately eight months after conception, his prognosis is excellent.

Summary

Obstetricians and students of fetal development arbitrarily divide the nine months of pregnancy into three equal units, the first, second and third trimester. To some extent this is an artificial division, for the baby grows progressively day by day with no abrupt change at any of these times. But this division into three equal periods is useful, for, as we have seen, certain characteristic changes generally occur within those time frames.

In the first trimester life gets started. The fertilized egg divides, becomes the morula and then the blastocyst which nestles into the mother's womb. It is a time of vigorous differentiation and formation of most of the structures that ultimately become the organs of the newborn child. The major activity of the fetus is directed, not toward growing larger, but in defining the roles of specialized cells and molding them into functioning organs. During this time, therefore, noxious agents can lead to organ malformations. They can produce birth defects such as deafness, blindness, mental retardation of certain types, heart malformations, cleft palate and lip and many others.

The second trimester is primarily geared toward growth in weight and size. Organ maturation does continue, and some hazards can cause injuries during this period, but for the most part the basic structures of the baby have already been formed. Environmental hazards and improper nutrition during the second trimester will not cause the same types of organ malformations as occur during the differentiation phase —the first trimester. Instead, they may produce organ malfunction, injury to already formed organs or impairment of body or organ growth. The result may be mental or physical retardation, weakened bodily defenses or other dysfunctions. We will elaborate upon these in much greater detail later when we consider specific hazards.

The last trimester is almost entirely a time of growth. During this period the baby most needs adequate and proper nutrition from his mother, including vitamins, iron, proteins to build his tissue structures, and fats and carbohydrates to fuel the fires that energize these growth processes. Poor maternal nutrition can retard this growth. Drugs and chemicals will not produce structural malformations of organs, but, just as in the second trimester, they may damage his tissues in other ways. His tissues are delicate, his defenses immature and his growing body and organs susceptible to injury.

Now we have witnessed the miraculous events of human reproduction. We have followed the baby's timetable and seen when and how important changes take place. Our next step is to understand how the baby relates to the outside world, so we know how we can favorably influence its environment. How does the baby get the nourishment it needs for proper growth and development? How do chemicals and drugs from the mother's system enter his body and invade those delicate, growing tissues? In the next chapter we explore the relationship of mother to child. We see how the growing baby is exposed to the outside world through its mother's body.

IV

The Placenta—Lifeline
Between Mother and Child

The cell is a remarkable self-contained unit that carries out all of the functions characteristic of life. It eats, breathes, burns fuel, repairs its broken parts and reproduces. An individual cell is minute—much too small to see with our naked eyes. Under a microscope it looks like a gelatinous blob with a flexible, balloon-like membrane containing its contents. The smallest living animals and plants—protozoa and bacteria—consist of a single cell. What a contrast between those tiny one-celled organisms and a human being whose body contains billions of cells packed together into special forms, each having unique functions!

Feeding the Cells

All cells share the same basic needs. They must be supplied with nutrients—the building blocks, the catalysts and the fuel—that they need to stay alive. They must have a constant source of oxygen to drive the internal power plants that burn the fuel. They must eliminate wastes that would otherwise accumulate and choke them to death. All of these exchanges of molecules (tiny particles) of foods, fuel, oxygen and wastes must go on continuously and instantaneously. In less time than it took to read these first paragraphs, each of your body's cells shuttled back and forth across its membrane boundaries thousands of such molecules.

The cells that form the growing child have special eating and breathing needs since they are in a state of constant activity. Dividing to make new cells, forming new tissues and new organs, growing larger at a breakneck pace takes lots of energy and materials. Yet the growing child can't eat as we do nor can she take a deep breath. How then does she get the food that she needs and the oxygen that her cells demand? How can she dispose of the wastes that remain from the fires burning inside her active cells?

Before birth, all cellular needs are provided by the mother through her bloodstream. When the mother breathes, she carries oxygen from the air around her into her lungs where it passes into her blood and to her growing child. Carbon dioxide made in the baby's active cells bubbles into mother's bloodstream and is swept to the lungs and out of her body when she exhales. Essential nutrients enter the mother's blood through her intestinal tract after she eats a meal. Among them are amino acids—the building blocks of proteins that form much of the cell's structure; sugar and fats—the vital fuels that provide the energy to power the cell's tireless activities, and vitamins—necessary chemicals which help the cell to properly carry out its chemical reactions. They, too, are pumped by the mother's heart through her arteries and into her uterus where they can get to the developing child. There they are gobbled up hungrily by the tireless growing cells. At the same time, chemical wastes are passed to the mother's blood for transport to the outside via the kidneys and out through her urine, or to be exhaled from her lungs.

This choppy description of the movement of nutrients, oxygen and wastes between mother and growing child can't do justice to the remarkable rapidity and smooth flow of these events. The back-and-forth movement is strikingly regular and uninterrupted, like waves lapping against the beach and rolling back again into the ocean. The growing baby and her mother interact through the mother's bloodstream without a moment's pause 24 hours a day for 266 days.

This interaction never stops but it does change as the child grows. As the individual progresses from a one-celled, fertilized ovum into a complex fetus containing millions of specialized cells, its requirements alter. The way that nutrients, gases and wastes are delivered in and out of the cells becomes increasingly complex. Since all of the chapters that follow deal with the movement of foods, chemicals, drugs and things good and bad from mother to child, you should have a picture of how this interaction works. The remainder of this chapter will describe that relationship and will lay the groundwork for things to come.

Nourishing the Growing Baby

If you recall from the previous chapter, the new baby starts life as a single cell which is fertilized, then divides into a grapelike cluster of many cells called the morula. The morula travels down the fallopian tube, steadily making its way toward the uterus. Like all cells, it needs nourishment and oxygen to complete its travels and to continue dividing. It gets these directly from fluid secreted by the mother's cells that line the fallopian tube. Because the morula is quite tiny, nutrients, oxygen, carbon dioxide and other wastes can pass directly through its surrounding membranes into and out of its cells. For simplification we will call this process of direct passage "diffusion."* Picture this like a sponge or a paper towel soaking up water. The water and dissolved materials pass directly into the pores and spaces of the towel or sponge. Like a sponge, cells can soak up fluid and its contents that surround them and can squeeze out carbon dioxide and chemical wastes that are building up inside.

Shortly after the morula enters the mother's uterus, it becomes the blastocyst. The blastocyst begins to dig and burrow its way into the tissues that line the moth-

*Readers with a scientific background will recognize that passage of nutrients and gases in and out of cells involves many additional and more complex processes such as active transport, pinocytosis, facilitated transport and others. For easier communication with a general audience we shall include all of these in the term "diffusion."

er's womb. Now nourishment and oxygen reach the blastocyst through the mother's bloodstream via tiny blood vessels that surround and bathe it in fluid.

For the first several weeks the growing embryo is sufficiently small to obtain its nourishment and eliminate its wastes by direct diffusion. Soon, however, the embryo becomes too large and too complex to exchange these chemicals this way. Its cells have expanded, twisted and folded into such an array that they are no longer reached and nourished by the fluids and blood in the mother's womb. Substances must find a new way to move in and out of this increasingly complex individual.

Now the baby's heart and bloodstream come into play. The heart pumps blood through the body of the growing child, delivering nutrients and oxygen to its innermost cells and returning wastes to its mother. Blood pumped by the baby's heart passes through large arteries, into smaller arteries, and finally into tiny capillaries, no larger than a single blood cell. The tiny capillaries come into direct contact with all of the growing baby's cells. Diffusion still takes place between those cells and the capillaries. Now, however, the baby uses its own bloodstream to get those materials where they need to go.

Thus the baby is beginning to do its part to move life-giving substances in and dangerous wastes out of its body. But the mother remains a vital link in this chain of chemical movement, for she is the connection to the outside world. Before anything can get to the baby, it must pass through the mother's bloodstream. Materials that are passed out of the fetus exit via the mother. This hookup between mother and fetus occurs in the placenta. There, the baby's and mother's bloodstreams come into close contact. The blood of the two never actually mix, but their pools of blood come so close that diffusion between them readily takes place.

The first phase of this specialized connection between mother and child appears almost as soon as the trophoblast burrows into the uterus. The relationship gradually becomes more and more complex and mature until it consists of the very sophisticated placenta and umbilical cord. The umbilical cord is the conduit which houses the large arteries and vein that whisk the baby's blood on the round trip from its body to the placenta and back. This connection between mother and child—the placenta and the umbilical blood vessels —is a miracle of nature and the hallmark of prenatal life. Since it is the route by which almost all materials, good and bad, get to the growing child, we shall discuss in some detail the placenta, its formation, function and structure. The purpose: to help you understand how the things you take into your body can reach and affect your child.

Formation of the Placenta

The formation of the placenta, its circulation and complex connection between mother and child, is a synchronized ballet involving many activities of many different cell types. For our purposes it will suffice to paint a general picture of this development, without delving into all the confusing details.

From the moment the blastocyst bores into its new home within its mother's uterus, preparation begins for the nine-month stay. We have already seen how rapidly cells begin to differentiate into their permanent functions; how organs begin to take shape; how many of the baby's structures are well on their way toward development before the embryo is an inch long. While all of this is taking place, other specialized cells move into action. Their job is to form the bridge that will connect the child to its mother—the critical contact between the child and the outside world (figure 1).

Small fingerlike arrays of cells stretch outward from the growing child and tap into the mother's womb. They begin as a central stalk which spreads and divides until it becomes a lacy network known as a villus (plural villi). It resembles an array of roots emanating from a single stem (on that weed that you pick from your garden, for example) (figure 1).

As these villi form, burrowing deeper and more widely into the mother's womb, the blood vessels that

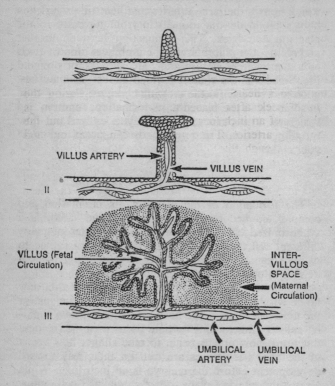

Figure 1 Growth of the Placenta
I. First bud of villus stalk
II. Forming villus containing new fetal blood vessels
III. Mature villi with rootlike configurations

course within them also take shape. Each tiny finger-like villus contains a single artery that will carry blood away from the baby, a single vein that will bring the blood back and a small capillary that connects the two.

Each of these villus arteries arises from one of two main umbilical arteries. These are the primary pipe-lines that lead out of the baby. Blood is pumped by the baby's heart (remember this begins during the fourth week after fertilization, when the embryo is only ⅜ of an inch long) through its body and out the umbilical arteries. The arteries divide, spread out and course through the villi to the very tips of the finger-like projections. There they transiently become the vil-lus capillaries, which make a hairpin turn and lead back into the villus veins. Those veins retrace the steps of the arteries and return to the villus stalk. Multiple veins merge until finally there is only one, the main umbilical vein. This single vessel that runs through the umbilical cord (there are two umbilical arteries) is the final connection between mother and child. It car-ries everything to the growing child that it needs for continued growth. This conglomeration of two umbilical arteries, villus arteries, villus capillaries, villus veins and umbilical vein is the fetal component of the pla-cental circulation. It is the route by which blood enters and leaves the baby, getting its nourishment and oxy-gen, and releasing its carbon dioxide and other wastes along the way.

To complete the placental circulation, the mother must do her part. Tiny uterine capillaries from the mother's circulation empty directly into the spaces between the villi known, logically, as intervillous spaces. Blood flows into those spaces and gradually out through other capillaries which lead into maternal veins. Eventually, as the villi become larger and more mature, and as the growing child requires greater supplies of food and oxygen, large maternal arteries empty directly into the intervillous spaces. These so-called "spiral arteries" forcefully propel blood into the intervillous spaces through the driving action of the mother's heart. Veins, now opening into the spaces,

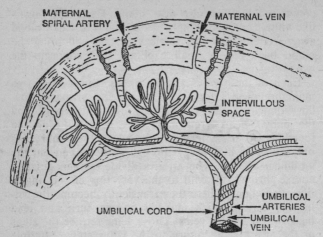

Figure 2   Mature Placenta and Umbilical Cord

drain the blood from the spaces and return it to the mother's lungs and heart. Thus, we have two discrete circulations in the placental unit: the fetal circulation which flows through the villi and back; the maternal circulation which pours blood into the intervillous spaces, surrounding the villi in a bath of life-giving fluid (figures 1 and 2).

The two circulations never mix directly. The fetal blood remains in its vessels confined by the membranes of the vessels themselves and the cells that line the surrounding villus sheath. The maternal blood percolates through the intervillous spaces confined by the villus membranes, never directly contacting the fetal blood. But the membranes are thin, and small chemicals, gases, nutrients, waste products and drugs can slip through and be transferred back and forth from mother to child. This occurs through the process of diffusion and related mechanisms that we mentioned earlier (figures 2 and 3).

The fetal and maternal circulations are the chief function of the placenta. But the placenta has other uses and components as well. These include a variety of structural tissues which give it its shape, form and

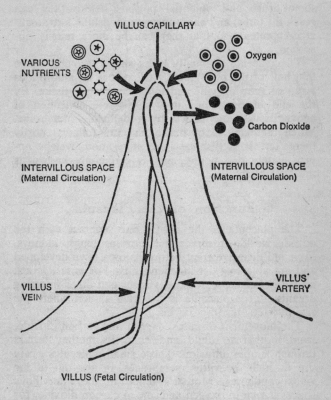

Figure 3 Villus tip enlarged many times to show blood vessels and movement of gases and nutrients from fetus to mother and mother to fetus.

individuality, and numerous metabolically active tissues that produce certain hormones, participate in transporting materials from mother to child, destroy some drugs and potential poisons before they can reach the fetus, and chop up some foodstuffs into smaller components so that they can be more readily absorbed.

The placenta gradually takes shape throughout the first half of the pregnancy. At first it is an amorphous array of growing villi and loose connective tissue. By the end of pregnancy it is a discrete collection of active tissues surrounded by a definable membrane. When the baby is born the placenta follows shortly thereafter. It is dishlike in configuration, weighs approximately one pound, and is commonly known as the "afterbirth."

Function of the Placenta

The placenta is the baby's only contact with the outside world. It serves the fetus as lungs, kidneys, liver and digestive tract before its own have developed and are able to exist independently. For gases, foods, hosts of chemicals, poisons, viruses and other infecting organisms, the placenta is the train station where the ride into fetal territory begins.

The movement of gases, oxygen and carbon dioxide, from mother to child and child to mother occurs through simple diffusion. Those small molecules easily slip through the villus membranes, in and out of the villus capillaries. Mother's blood in the intervillous spaces is rich in oxygen and low in carbon dioxide; for it recently passed through her lungs where oxygen was breathed in and carbon dioxide exhaled. The baby's villus capillary blood, on the other hand, is rich in carbon dioxide and low in oxygen. The placenta, you see, is the last stop. Fetal blood gets there only after it traverses the baby's body where cells take in the oxygen and deposit their carbon dioxide waste. Laws of diffusion force molecules to move from sites where their concentration is high to sites where it is low. This sets the stage for the proper and necessary transfer of gases between maternal and fetal circulations. The mother's oxygen-rich intervillous blood pours oxygen molecules into the oxygen-poor villus capillaries. The overloaded fetal blood deposits its carbon dioxide waste into the intervillous pool and the maternal circulation. In this way the blood that returns to the fetus has been enriched with oxygen and stripped of much of its carbon dioxide. This movement is pictured in figure 3.

Most foods and nutrients move in somewhat more complex ways. Diffusion still plays some role, but other processes such as active transport assist the amino acids, some vitamins, carbohydrates and fats in their passage from mother to child. But the principle is the same. They move from a region of high concentration into a nutrient-poor one where they are needed. In this case, the mother's intervillous blood is loaded with nutritious substances, absorbed from her intestinal tract after she eats a meal. The baby's villus capillary blood is devoid of most nutrients since they were deposited in its tissues during the rounds of the child's body. The movement, then, is in the expected direction—mother to child (figure 3).

A great many drugs, viruses, poisons from the atmosphere, and chemical food additives can pass into the baby as readily as foods and gases—something we have learned quite recently. Scientists used to believe that there was a so-called "placental barrier" —a kind of an armed fortress that differentiated between good things and bad, letting the good things pass while barring the bad ones. It is true that some substances are destroyed by the placenta and that others are unable to get through. But many things that we would like to keep out slip through easily. For those drugs and chemicals that have been studied, the "placental barrier" is more like a wide-holed sieve: the vast majority pass effortlessly into the baby. As we will see later, many of these intruders are staunch fetal enemies.

Now we have seen how the baby grows and how

she comes in contact with the outside world through her mother. Let's move on to her chemical environment. What good nutrients and vital materials do you need to give her? Which ones should you try to keep out?

Section Two
NUTRITION

V

Care and Feeding of the Growing Baby

"I'm pregnant again, and I'm as confused as ever about proper diet. What should I eat and how much? Is there anything I should avoid or be sure to get enough of? Can I gain as much weight as I want to, or should I struggle to fight the pounds? One friend says one thing, another something else. Even our doctors don't agree."

It's hard to get the right answers. No topic has been more distorted by folklore, fad mongers and man's imagination than how to feed the pregnant woman. From liquid diets to pasty goo; from non-caloric meals to extra-high-energy fatty concoctions; from bland, tasteless foods to highly spiced fare; six bananas a day; two gallons of milk; kelp and yeast—all these have been, at various times and in various places the staples for pregnant women. Yet, as varied as these diets might be, they share a common heritage—the belief that pregnant women are somehow different, and that they deserve special handling. And that's the truth— pregnant women do have special needs.

What you, as a pregnant woman, don't need is a barrage of contradictory recommendations. You've got enough trouble with fatigue, morning sickness, and heartburn. Fortunately, there are some simple rules of good eating for you to follow, but first we must break through some of the folklore that still lingers. Even in twentieth-century America, "experts," official or self-styled, can make your head spin utterly bewildered. All of you who have shared pregnancy gossip know what we mean.

"My doctor says I shouldn't gain more than two pounds a month."

"Well, mine says it's all right to gain four pounds, but only after the fourth month."

"I'm scared to death. If I gain more than eighteen pounds my doctor says he might not deliver the baby because he can't be responsible for the consequences."

"My obstetrician is just great! He says I can eat as much as I want to. The baby needs the food. Whatever weight I gain is fine."

You can be sure of one thing: they can't all be right. The fact is that many of these dogmas arise from folk myths spawned by society and canonized by physicians. Most physicians and most cultures from the early Greeks to modern-day Manhattanites have set arbitrarily low limits for weight gain in pregnancy.

From pimples to strokes, every imaginable malady of mother and child has been ascribed, at one time or another, to excessive weight gain. Most of these tales sprang from the fancy of folk healers and story tellers. However, not too long ago, there was one risk that was a real danger to be reckoned with.

The pelvis, the group of bones that connects your legs to the rest of your body, forms a narrow passageway through which the baby must pass to reach its new world. In the eighteenth century many women had abnormally narrow pelvises due to general malnutrition and rickets (vitamin D deficiency) which was widespread in the new urban centers.[1] The journey through the pelvis to the outside is the most perilous adventure in our lives. If the baby is too large, or the pelvis too narrow, the infant will get stuck on the way out. The result can be disastrous: death or severe injury for the baby and often for the mother.

Physicians of the eighteenth century recognized this hazard and embraced the only logically available solution—smaller babies. How could the babies be kept small? Simple. By feeding the mothers less. This answer did help solve the immediate problem. The number of birth injuries was reduced, since restricting food during pregnancy did make smaller babies and easier egress out of the mother. But this dietary manipulation had its price. Smaller babies were less resistant to disease. They were often sickly, malformed and vulnerable to fatal infections and other maladies that awaited them. Their chances of dying after birth were, therefore, high. What's more, even if they survived, their likelihood of achieving full mental and physical development was lessened by undernutrition before birth.

Large babies no longer pose the threat they once did. Rickets is rare in this country, and women's pelvises are wider. And for those that are still too narrow to accommodate the baby, modern medicine can help. Special diagnostic studies such as sonography and X-ray pelvimetry can tell doctors just what size the pelvis is. They can help predict the chances for safe vaginal delivery. If things aren't right, improved anesthesia and surgical techniques enable a safe operative delivery. Cesarean section, the operation that pulls the baby directly out of the mother's abdomen, makes it unnecessary to force that big baby through a narrow pelvis. As a result, dieting to keep babies small is a relic of the past, like biting on a bullet while the surgeon cuts, and having leeches suck one's blood to get rid of the "bad humors." These days the small risk of having a large baby can't compare with the lifelong threat of poor prenatal nutrition.

Old-time bans on weight gain were sparked by real concerns about delivery complications, but they were fueled by a widely held misconception. Everyone—physicians, scientists, mothers-to-be—believed that the deck was always stacked in favor of the growing fetus. Somehow this creature would always come out on top. Even though his mother might diet, we could count on him to be a successful parasite feeding greedily and well from his mother's tissues and "reserves."

We now know that this just isn't so. Certainly the fetus can tap some nourishment, particularly calories, from its mother's stores, but not enough to support proper growth and development. What's more, though she might give up some fat that's lying around, she doesn't have any extra supply of proteins. They're all tied up in her vital organs. If she had to give up any, she would have to donate them from her heart, liver, lungs, brain or muscles. Quite obviously she couldn't spare even small pieces of those high-protein organs. The upshot is that the growing baby must be supplied with nutrients of his own. A mother must eat enough of the right types of foods to supply her continuing needs and to feed her very hungry unborn child.

Now that we know that prenatal nutrition is important, we move to the next logical questions. By now you may be asking "How can we tell if a newborn is undernourished?" "Can a mother change this by improving her diet?" and "Is it really known that apparent undernourishment at birth means poor performance in later life?"

One of the best tests of the state of maternal nutrition is found in the birth weight of her offspring. Good maternal nutrition before and during pregnancy, particularly the last trimester, in general, produces larger babies.[2-7] For example:

Children of low socioeconomic groups in which nutrition is marginal are smaller than babies born to affluent members of the same society.[3]

Dutch babies born during the famine of World War II were considerably smaller than those born later or earlier. Furthermore, their birth weights were quite dependent on when they were exposed to the famine. Those whose mothers were undernourished during the last trimester of pregnancy were the smallest.[5, 8]

The birth weights of poor Indians from Guatemala can be increased by providing pregnant women with high-protein, high-caloric diets.[2, 3]

To be sure, nutrition is not the only answer. There are other critical determinants of birth weight, and often it is most difficult to isolate nutrition's role. Racial background, genetic makeup, and maternal size are other important factors. Thus North American Indian children whose mother's diets are protein-poor but high in calories are the largest of any babies. Their average birth weight is 7½ pounds.[9] Is this genetically directed, or is it due to the nature of the calories in the diet, or to some other unknown factor? We really don't have the answer. We do know that most undernourished peoples suffer from both protein and caloric malnutrition. We also know that their babies are small and that improved feeding makes them larger. A group like the American Indians must be judged on their own scale. Thus, a 7-pound Indian infant might be seriously undernourished, whereas his Caucasian counterpart would be considered normal.

The conclusion, then, is that birth weight is one index of nutritional status that must be evaluated in its proper context. It is not absolute or a sole determinant of good health. There are many exceptions among different societies and among individuals within the same society. But it is a useful relative guide to be considered along with other factors. Quite frequently, when nutrition is poor within a group of people, this will be reflected in low birth weights.

Does birth weight matter? Does it make any difference if the children are small? When low birth weight is due to maternal undernutrition, birth weight appears to matter a great deal. Many studies have suggested that there is a relationship between birth weight and later performance. Low birth weight children do not, in general, fare as well as their larger counterparts.* Low birth weight is associated with a higher infant mortality, congenital deformities, poor growth and development and intellectual blunting.[10-20] Here are just a few examples:

The average birth weight in one large group of mentally retarded children was considerably lower than normal.[10]

*Please note that we keep saying "in general." We do this because there are many individual exceptions, and we don't want to leave you with the false impression that low birth weight automatically means a future of trouble. It is merely one guide that has some meaning when applied to large populations. If you ate well, but your child's birth weight was low simply because you are a small person, there is probably no cause for concern. If, on the other hand, your diet was poor, the low birth weight of your child takes on greater significance.

A large English study involving 15,000 school children found that severe handicaps, including mental retardation, cerebral palsy, mongolism and a variety of birth defects were far more common in children whose birth weights fell far below average.[21]

Very interesting and meaningful studies involving twins have shown that, in general, the child with the larger birth weight fared better both mentally and physically.[22] This type of study may be the best test of the effects of nutrition and birth weight, since it tends to eliminate other variables such as environmental and socioeconomic forces. After all, these children grow up in the same family.

We may be witnessing a frightening effect of the fad for reduced birth weights. In this country, one of the most prosperous and medically sophisticated in the world, our infant mortality rate is shockingly high. We rank only sixteenth among Western countries at keeping our children alive. Some have postulated that this may be due, in part, to our fetish for unhealthy dietary restrictions in pregnancy.[23] By vigorously fighting weight gain, American mothers may be threatening the very survival of their babies. Starvation in the midst of plenty—self-imposed at that—may be the silent killer of many American infants.

In all fairness, we must point out that not all authorities agree that birth weight and prenatal nutrition are vital factors in future potential. They cite the vast interplay of social, economic, genetic, environmental and other influences as matters of major importance. In general, those who don't embrace nutrition theories have no major criticism of the role of nutrition. They merely believe that other elements are equally or, at times, more important. We agree wholeheartedly. For instance, in one study which compared the intellectual progress of 19-year-olds who had been starved before birth during the Dutch famine and were born small, there was a better correlation between social class and intellectual achievement than there was between birth weight and mental capability.[24] It may well be that environmental influences, such as home stimulation, better feeding later, freedom from diseases of overcrowding, were able to compensate for a great deal of the harm done by early starvation. Undeniably, later events play a major role in development. But this sort of observation should not divert our attention away from the importance of prenatal nutrition. The studies above, particularly the follow-up of twins having different weights, is an inescapable clue that nutrition before birth and birth weight are relevant.

A vivid analogy might help to put prenatal nutrition and birth weight in proper perspective. Suppose a builder has a pile of wood that is full of knots and badly warped. Can he build a good house from these materials? If the architecture is well planned, the other materials of high quality, the general workmanship good, these can compensate for the imperfections of those structural elements. The undernourished baby, like that wood, is born with innate warpage. Sure, hard work, proper training, an ideal environment may overcome many of the deficiencies. But isn't it better to start with strong raw materials?

Does this mean that Alice, your new baby, who weighed only six pounds, is destined for a life of problems and catching up; that she won't match your heavier first child or eight-pound Billy down the street? Not necessarily, for there are many individual considerations (see footnote 1). If your health is good, and the foods you ate before and during pregnancy well-balanced, there will probably be no problems with Alice. Also, if you are small, the "normal" size for your baby may be considerably less than that of your two-hundred-pound neighbor's baby. But when birth weights are reduced by poor prenatal nutrition, those children will have more problems than the babies of well-fed mothers.

Another measurement that correlates with birth weight, prenatal nutrition and future achievement is head circumference.[2, 25] The circumference of a newborn's head is a number that can easily be assessed by placing a tape measure around in a standard fashion. It is roughly correlated with brain size—the larger the brain, theoretically, the greater the intellectual potential (though this has not been proven with absolute certainty). Very recently scientists have begun to understand why prenatal nutrition is so important to brain growth and, hence, to likely future mental performance.

If you remember, all of the organs of the body were nearly fully formed by the time the fetus was two months old. At that point, it was only 1½ inches long. Quite obviously, an exceptional amount of growth of these organs must go on after that point to produce a life-sized baby. Organs and tissues grow by two means. First, cells may divide and make new cells. This is called hyperplasia. Second, cells may merely accumulate additional fluid, protein, and other chemicals. They swell and become larger—in a sense getting fatter—but they don't increase in number. This is called hypertrophy. If every cell in an organ were to become twice as fat as before, the net effect would be to double the size of that organ, even though no new cells were added.

All tissues and organs of the growing fetus grow by hyperplasia (cell division) throughout gestation. Hypertrophy (cell fattening) comes into play in later months and at different times for different organs. Thus, the liver probably contains its full complement of cells—the number that it will have for the rest of the person's life—by the time the child is born. It will continue to enlarge into adulthood, but mainly by cell hypertrophy. The brain, on the other hand, continues to make new cells in addition to swelling by cell hypertrophy from its first appearance at two to three weeks of embryonic age until at least one year after birth. However, the rate of cell division and, hence, new cell formation, is much greater before birth than it is later. A great fear among embryologists, nutritionists and pediatricians which has held up under experimental scrutiny, is that prenatal nutritional deficiency will lead to a permanent loss of brain cells which can never, even by good feeding after birth, be regained. Those cells that weren't made *in utero* are lost forever. The result: likely reduction in intellectual capacity. Rather sophisticated studies of brain cell number, head circumference and their relationship to prenatal nutrition and to later achievement tend to bolster this supposition.[21, 26-29]

One large-scale study among American poor warned that even here, where nutrition is relatively good, millions of youngsters may bear the permanent scars of undernutrition before birth. In a population of middle-class Americans, the vast majority were born with good-sized heads. Only three percent were far below the usual normal. In a group of thousands of poverty-level youngsters, however, the results were quite different. Seventeen percent were born with heads far below the general circumference. The investigator concluded that as many as two million children born annually in this country risk impaired brain development.[25]

Another fascinating study, in a related but different vein, has recently added support for the belief that poor prenatal nutrition, particularly early in gestation, may permanently impair aspects of brain development. The observation arose from a clever and careful survey of a unique group of people. These were victims of a short-lived drastic famine in the Netherlands between November 1944 and May 1945, the Nazi retaliation for the resistance movement. Children who were exposed to that famine during the first six months of intrauterine development stood a far greater chance of becoming obese later in life than those whose mothers were adequately nourished during that phase of pregnancy. The suggested explanation was that malnutrition during that critical period of brain development impaired the growth of that part of the brain that controls eating and weight gain. Because that region, the hypothalamus, was imperfectly formed, the scientists theorized, normal controls of eating patterns went awry.[8] The result was overeating and obesity.

Although this study was most interested in mechanisms of adult obesity, it gives us a very important message about the role of prenatal nutrition in the growth and development of the brain. It illustrates the possible adverse effect of early malnutrition on brain growth. Surely if the region of the brain that controls eating can be affected, other essential brain sites must suffer as well.

Low birth weight and small head circumference may bode ill for future mental and physical achievement. In addition, poor prenatal nutrition may bring scores of other problems. The effects of maternal undernutrition vary widely—failure of conception or implantation, frequent miscarriages, birth defects, gross physical and mental deficiencies, death shortly after birth or subtle defects in physical or intellectual growth which may never be recognized—are some that have been identified or considered.[14-18, 30-33] Let us look at some of these other dangers.

Procreation is not abolished by a society's malnutrition. A brief glance at the poorest underdeveloped nations, buried under an avalanche of new people, tells us that. However, their poor nutrition does reduce the fertility rate and it does increase the chances for miscarriages. This means that more sexual encounters and more pregnancies are required to produce each child. Moreover, the children of those malnourished mothers are off to a very bad start.

And what about the "affluent" West? Recall the study that warned of stunted head size and probable brain growth impairment among American poor.[25] Keep in mind, too, that "good nutrition" is a relative term. When we compare the nutritional value in the junk foods of our American youngsters with the sparse fare of a poor African tribe, our kids are better nourished. But would well-balanced meals and supplemental vitamins better prepare them for motherhood? The answer is an unqualified, yes!

It is now well established that the basic nutritional needs of teenagers are greater than those of young adults. This is undoubtedly due to the special demands that this time of growth and maturation places upon them. When they become pregnant, these demands are heightened even further. Unfortunately, teenage American girls neglect their nutritional needs at a time when they need the most support. If they become pregnant during this period, or shortly after they leave their teens, they often provide an environment for the un-born child which is far from optimal.[34-37] Young wom-en must begin preparing nutritionally for motherhood well in advance of the time they actually become pregnant.

We have noted the relatively high perinatal mor-tality rate in this country and the small birth weight and head circumference of less-well-nourished new-borns. We have considered how these deficiencies affect mental and physical performance in later life. In most cases, in our society, the effects are subtle. The children may not be grossly deformed or sickly like starving youngsters in India, but they may never achieve their full potentials. This is the greatest scourge of undernu-trition in Western societies since it strikes silently, eludes detection, but undercuts the very strength and fiber of society.

We all have high hopes for our children. We wish them good health, happiness, success, intelli-gence. Many ingredients working together mold the final outcome of their lives and determine whether or not these goals are achieved. We can control some of those ingredients, others we cannot.

The component over which we have the least con-trol is our genetic programming—the code words and messages that we pass to our children. True, today geneticists are tapping the surface of genetic counsel-ing. They can tell us how likely we are to transmit certain diseases like sickle cell anemia, hemophilia and Huntington's chorea. But for every genetic risk that can be avoided or altered through counseling, millions of others cannot. Thus, for the most part, we are slaves to our genes. We work within the limits imposed by them. They tell us who we are.

Within the boundaries of our genetic capabilities, we have wide latitude. Our genes may tell us how far we can ultimately go, but other factors spur us on or hold us back.[38] Socioeconomic backgrounds, early up-bringing, parental attitudes, education and, at the top of the list, nutrition, play a great role in the develop-ment of the full person. The greatest worry in this country is not gross, obvious malnutrition that brings to mind pictures of babies with swollen bellies or people dying in the streets. No, the greatest worries are the subtle restraints that imperfect nutrition may bring. What a shame if our children never achieve their full potentials because they started life in a poor nutritional environment.

When is the right time to begin the program of good eating? Ample studies have now shown that the mother's nutritional status before she becomes pregnant is at least as important, if not more important, than what she eats during pregnancy. Actually, there are three crucial phases in the nutritional environment of the young child: the nutritional status of his mother before he was even conceived; the nine months of intrauterine growth, particularly the last four; and the first year or so after birth when brain growth is still active.

In simple terms, your nutritional status before and during your pregnancy mean a great deal to your child. A lifelong program of well-balanced nutrition, including adequate calories, wholesome proteins, vitamins, minerals and salts gives the child the best possible start in life. It doesn't guarantee a productive or healthy future, but it starts him in that direction. There is no place for rigorous dieting in pregnancy. You should eat full, well-balanced meals. You should aim for a weight gain of 22 to 27 pounds.[34] The next chapter will give you some practical modern hints about how and what to eat during pregnancy and before you become pregnant.

VI

A Guide to Daily Diet
for the Pregnant Woman

Rules of good eating are twice as important when you are pregnant. You are eating for two, and your growing baby is particularly greedy. The vitamins, minerals, fats, carbohydrates, calories and amino acid building blocks that make the protein structures of her new body all come from you. So, even if you never before paid much attention to what you popped into your mouth, now that you're thinking about getting pregnant or have already taken the step it's time to start noticing what you eat. "It's my body. I'll do what I want to with it," won't do any more.

Most Americans are appallingly uninterested in nutrition. You probably chose your outfit today more carefully than you chose your breakfast. Even many physicians are surprisingly uninformed and unconcerned about nutrition. They come from medical schools which until recently didn't even mention the word "nutrition," let alone teach a course in it. Most seventh graders fresh out of their home economics classes know more about foods than many physicians. Unfortunately, most of those seventh graders promptly forget or brush aside whatever worthwhile tips they have acquired.

The Well-Balanced Diet

We grew up, as probably most of you did, believing that "The usual American diet is well balanced" and "If you eat regular meals with portions from each of the basic categories—meat and meat substitutes, milk and milk products, breads and cereal, fruits and vegetables—you'll get all of the nutrients you need."

We also believed that vitamin supplements were extravagant and unnecessary if our meals were "well balanced." Maybe so, but the "average American diet" today is probably never "well balanced"; thus, vitamin and mineral supplements may be needed unless you very carefully plan your meals.

You know how much transportation, communication, and automation have changed in the last fifty years. Well, food production, processing and preparation have seen far more radical alterations in the past ten. Perhaps ten or twenty years ago there was a "well-balanced" American diet. Now it is buried under the bags, cans, boxes and jars of junk and processed foods on our supermarket shelves. Try as you may, it is probably impossible to resurrect those balanced diets.

Breads and cereals certainly aren't what they used to be. Milling, bleaching, processing, refining destroy vitamins, and strip away fiber and protein. The bread and cereal that was an important part of yesterday's well-balanced diet doesn't give us what bread and cereal is supposed to.

The same is true for processed, canned, frozen and pasteurized fruits, vegetables, juices and dairy products. Some may retain full food value, some part, some very little. The problem is that you as consumer and concerned pregnant woman never know which is which. Eating those prepared foods is like playing dinner-table Russian roulette. Here's a shocking example. A recent article in the *Journal of the American Medical Association* evaluated the vitamin C content and activity of frozen and pasteurized orange juices.[1] If you are like us, you've probably always believed that the morning glass of orange juice was a wholesome member of that fruit-and-vegetable category. Probably many of you thought, as we did, "Here's our vitamin C for the day."

Well, we've been wrong. It turns out that most of our canned fruit juices have lost a good deal of their active vitamin C. It's destroyed in the pasteurization process. And for years this has been the vitamin C source for most of our "balanced" American diets. This discovery is most upsetting, and the implications go far beyond vitamin C alone. It makes us wonder what other nutritional deficiencies modern processing might be bringing. It took years before the effect of pasteurization on juices was uncovered. How long before we learn what else we are missing?

Add to food processing our modern cooking methods, and we've really lost touch with that ideal "balanced diet." High-temperature baking, boiling, deep-frying, pressure-cooking, and microwaving. What do these miracles of today's kitchens do to improve nutrients? Perhaps nothing. Perhaps a great deal. We really don't know.

The inescapable conclusion is that today's foods aren't what they used to be. If you pick and choose your foods very carefully, you may not need many supplements. If not, vitamin or mineral pills may have to become part of the morning routine. Before you can decide if and how to supplement your diet, you need to know what nutrients are essential, how much you and your unborn child need, and what foods contain them. First, what nutrients do you need and how much?

The Right Answers
About Nutritional Needs

There are two warring factions, each of which thinks it knows the answers. First, the official study group of the Federal Government, The Food and Nutrition Board of the National Academy of Sciences–National Research Council (from here on we'll call them the NRC for short). They are the ones who promulgate the Recommended Dietary Allowances (RDA)—the numbers that appear on cereal boxes. The arm of that organization that is concerned with maternal and prenatal nutrition is fittingly called the "Committee on Maternal Nutrition."

On the other side of the conflict lie the food faddists and fanatic proponents of unproved and untested high-dose mineral and vitamin supplementation. Let us briefly consider each side, then try to sort out some semblance of truth and good sense. Perhaps we then can arrive at reasonable recommendations for you.

Although they may be imprecise, the recommendations by the NRC are about the best we have today. Unfortunately, those RDA's—vitamins, minerals, etc., —have become, in the eyes of some people, sacred numbers that can never be questioned. Actually, many are derived in a very primitive way. They represent the amounts of nutrients that are needed to stave off gross and serious deficiency states, with a bit extra thrown in for good measure. Thus the recommended allowance of vitamin C will keep our gums and tissues from rotting away with scurvy. If we eat the amount of vitamin D that is recommended we won't become victims of rickets. The stipulated quantities of thiamine (vitamin B_1) and niacin will ward off beriberi and pellagra. "Enough" iron and folic acid will keep us from becoming anemic, and so forth and so on.

We know very little about the less obvious effects of vitamin and mineral undernutrition—impaired resistance, susceptibility to specific diseases, premature aging, etc.—though many of these questions have been touched upon or are under current scrutiny by scientists. The RDA's of the NRC may not be adequate to satisfy some of those subtle, still-undefined needs, but they represent the best and most current thinking. There is no good reason to consume more than the NRC tells us to. In many cases overzealous use of supplemental vitamins and minerals may be risky for you and your unborn child.

Vitamins occupy the center of the nutritional controversy, but other lesser-known and even less-well-understood dietary essentials have lined up on the battlefield. Did you know that there rages today a controversy about some trace minerals that you may never have heard about—cobalt, zinc, manganese, selenium, and chromium? Many scientists think we need these in our diets, perhaps a good deal more than we normally get, but equally learned authorities disagree. You can be sure that arguments about these trace minerals, and extravagant claims about their miraculous qualities, will soon take their place alongside the vitamin bottles.

The NRC recommendations must be recognized for what they are, not inviolate proclamations from Heaven, but rough guides that are derived from our still primitive understanding of nutrition.

In the hope of finding nutritional miracles many people turn to the faddists and purveyors of magic diets and megavitamin cures. For the most part, these recommendations are less accurate than those of the NRC. Generally they are derived from anecdotal experiences: sufferers from a malady who relate miracle cures allegedly brought about by a particular nutritional supplement. Many of those anecdotes have been tested by sophisticated laboratory studies, and most don't hold up. Vitamin E for vascular problems and impotency, and vitamin B_{12} for that "run-down feeling" are some examples.

The danger of such nutritional excesses is that vitamins and minerals taken in massive dosages become drugs. They are no longer natural body components, but are excess chemicals that must be disposed of or stored. We will learn in detail later that no drugs are safe in pregnancy. This applies to outrageous dosages of vitamins and minerals. Some can probably be taken with relative safety since they are water-soluble, and excesses are quickly shuttled out of the body through the urine. Others, including vitamins A, D, K, potassium and calcium, are clearly dangerous and must not be downed indiscriminately.

The message, then, is that our knowledge about proper nutrition is incomplete. Probably the correct answers lie somewhere in neutral territory, between the recommendations of the NRC and the food faddists. Or, even more likely, needs may vary markedly from individual to individual. But they are certainly increased in pregnancy.

The NRC tells us how much of each essential nutrient is needed for good health and the proper development of the unborn child. It also assures us that vitamin supplements are not necessary if our diets are "well balanced." This is probably true if you can make a very special effort to find that "well-balanced" diet in today's world of quick snacks and convenience foods. However, if you don't follow the type of diet that we recommend in table 2 but eat the usual fare of processed, canned, pasteurized and refined foods, you'll probably need some vitamin help. Stay away from fad diets and massive vitamin supplements. Most do no good, and some may be harmful to you or your baby.

Recommended Requirements

In the following paragraphs we will describe the quantities and types of foods, vitamins, proteins, minerals and calories that are generally recommended for you during pregnancy. While the future may bring changes, as we learn more about nutrition, these recommendations are up to date. When followed carefully they have produced healthy generations of American youngsters.

Proteins

Proteins are complex chemicals that serve two functions. First, they form the basic supporting tissues—cell membranes, connective tissue, muscle fibers, hair, etc.—that hold us together. Second, they serve as enzymes which speed up our chemical reactions so that we continue functioning efficiently. Proteins are obviously important to our well-being, and they are especially vital to the growing child who is building new tissue and carrying out reactions at a frantic pace.

Proteins are composed of chemical substructures known as amino acids. A total of 24 amino acids form the building blocks for all proteins. Our protein diets must be well balanced, since some sources of protein have more or less of certain amino acids. In particular, there are eight so-called essential amino acids which can only be found in adequate amounts in animal proteins. Thus, total vegetarian diets with no meats, milk or eggs are deficient. Vegetables, even when beans and nuts are included, lack enough of these essential amino acids. Growing fetuses whose sole source of amino acids comes from vegetables begin life with weakened tissues.

Some amino acids are damaged by pasteurization; thus pasteurized milk may not contain a full complement of protein builders. Fish, meats, and eggs, however, are excellent sources of most amino acids. They are complete animal proteins. Moreover, normal cooking does not significantly destroy their amino acids.

The daily requirement of protein increases in pregnancy. The nonpregnant woman needs only 46 grams or so daily. That second mouth to feed increases the requirement to 70 to 80 grams. To give you some idea what this means in real terms, a glass of milk has about 8 grams, a serving of meat or fish 15 to 40 grams (depending on leanness and size), and an egg, 6 grams. Thus four glasses of milk, one egg and one average 3- or 4-ounce (after cooking weight) portion of meat or fish preferably twice a day or substituted at one meal with another dairy dish such as yogurt or cheeses, plus the proteins found in cereal, bread, fruits and vegetables will provide the full supply of 70–80 grams. See tables 1 to 3.

Calories

For most Americans, getting enough calories poses very little problem. The greater difficulty is seeing to it that enough of the calories come from nutritious food such as those that contain proteins. A calorie, for those of you who have heard the word your whole lives but never knew what it meant, is a measure of energy. It represents the amount of energy that we can get out of a particular food when we burn it as fuel. All foods, including fats, carbohydrates and proteins, give up calories when they are burned, but only some foods find their major use in supplying calories for energy. Proteins, as we noted before, make up the form and the enzymes of the body. Consequently, even though proteins can be burnt for energy, we would rather put them to better use. Burning proteins would be like burning up the rafters of our houses one by one to keep us warm in the winter. Certainly we could get some warmth this way, but we would ultimately lose out—we would be homeless and colder than ever.

The major source of the calories that give our bodies energy and power, the tireless engines of the growing baby, comes from carbohydrates and fats.

The pregnant woman should consume at least 2400 calories. The amount, however, can go higher, depending upon the activities, both occupational and recreational, that you engage in. The more calories you expend, the more you will have to take in to supply your continued needs and the needs of the growing child. It's not hard to take in 2400 calories. Three full meals easily take care of that.

But remember the point we discussed in the previous chapter: pregnancy is no time to lose weight. Dieting and strict limitation of caloric intake are wrong for the pregnant woman. But before you think, "Aha, now I can drink all the milk shakes and eat all the snacks I want," let us make one thing clear. Too much food, too many calories, massive weight gain aren't good either. It's not healthful for you or your baby to eat 4500 calories worth of junk and to gain 45 pounds in pregnancy. If you take in enough calories, along with substantial proteins, to gain 22 to 27 pounds during those nine months, you've struck a happy, healthful balance.

Fats

Fats contribute, with carbohydrates, to the burnable calories that can be used for fuel. In fact, per gram, they give off more energy and are, therefore, more potent sources of fuel. For the same reason, if they are eaten in larger quantities than they are expended, they quickly add to the burgeoning waistline. Fats are potent energy sources and also potent obesity makers.

Fats have other uses besides burnable fuel. Certain fats help, along with proteins, to make the membranes and structures of the body's cells. Others help the digestive tract to absorb certain essential vitamins. Many weight-conscious women try very hard to eliminate fats from their diets. During pregnancy this is not a good practice. Whole milk, rather than skim, and vegetable oil in cooking and salad dressings supply vital fat nutrients. They also contain high concentrations of vitamins A, D, E and K, which are soluble in fats and are important to you and your growing child.

Vitamins

Vitamins are chemicals that are found in various foods, cannot be made by the human body (therefore they must be eaten) and are essential participants in a wide variety of chemical reactions and physiologic processes. Many of the B vitamins help cells to burn sugars; vitamin A forms the pigment in the eyes that permit us to see; vitamin D helps us absorb and use the calcium and phosphorus we need for healthy teeth and bones; vitamin B_{12}, vitamin B_6 and folic acid help develop and support our red blood cells that carry the oxygen throughout the body. They also help keep our nervous tissues in good working order. Vitamin E protects cells from the destructive forces of chemical and environmental oxidants that would otherwise attack and break down many of our body's cells.

There are many other vitamins with many other uses, but this helps give some idea of the diversity, the wide range of important functions that vitamins serve. In a sense they are so different that they really shouldn't be classified together. They each have entirely unique purposes, peculiar daily requirements, different structures and properties. Their only similarity is that they don't fit into any other category. They are not fats, proteins or carbohydrates, but they are necessary to good nutrition. They have, thus been lumped together in a strange marriage under the common name, "vitamin."

If these tiny, seemingly passive molecules only knew what furious controversies and bitter battles they've created! No substances in the world have been the subjects of more theories, arguments, and knock-down-drag-out conflicts. Everyone is an expert, from the researchers at the NRC to the self-styled nutritionists, to the megavitamin therapists, to every mother who has her pet vitamin uses, cures, and "proper" daily regimes. This disarray of thought is due to the aura of mystery that has always surrounded these strange substances, and to our understandable desire for miracle cures. Vitamins have become the panacea and hope for good health of a great many Americans.

Most of the wondrous things that large doses of vitamins are supposed to do—from curing varicose veins, to preventing gas pains, irregularity, fatigue, sterility, miscarriages and thousands of others—have never been proven. When they are subjected to careful testing, one by one, these glowing claims generally collapse.

This isn't to say that vitamins aren't necessary to stave off gross deficiency states, nor would we be so presumptuous to claim that we have all of the answers about them. No, undoubtedly there is a great deal to learn, and the future may bring new and better recommendations. For now, however, the most accurate estimates of vitamin needs are the figures put out by the NRC (table 1). Outrageously high recommendations, such as 25,000 units of vitamin A per day, are nutritional quackery. Not only is this unnecessary, but it is quite dangerous—some people have died from prolonged overdoses of vitamin A of this magnitude.

B Vitamins

The recommended allowances of each of these is given in Table 1. They come from a wide variety of animal and vegetable sources but particularly from liver, whole unrefined grains, leafy vegetables, milk and eggs. Cooking and refining destroys many of them, so to be sure you get enough of each of them you should either take vitamin supplements that provide the amounts recommended in Table 1 or see to it that you get enough from foods that have been fortified or are unrefined and whose vitamin contents are delineated on the labels. Since, in today's world of food refinement and overzealous cooking, it's hard to be certain that you get enough from your food, it makes some sense to supplement your daily diet with a multivitamin tablet. For example, a recent study found that vitamin B_6 levels were unusually low in over 50 percent of normal pregnant American women with so-called "well-balanced, average American diets."[2] This kind of observation, like the vitamin C study of frozen orange juice mentioned earlier, suggests the need for vitamin supplementation, but only enough to meet the RDA of the NRC. In the case of the B vitamins, overdoses may be harmless, since they are water-soluble and are readily excreted in the urine. But even so, we can't be sure of their safety. In one case, some infants whose mothers took large quantities of vitamin B_6 during pregnancy were born with convulsive disorders. It was learned that the babies had developed a dependency on this vitamin, much as a drug addict becomes dependent on heroin. They needed special care and gradual weaning from their vitamin B_6 "habit" to save their lives. Thus, even a seemingly harmless vitamin may not be so harmless to the unborn child. Vitamins in massive quantities become drugs, and most drugs are not safe in pregnancy.[3]

Vitamin A

This is found in milk, liver, dark-green and yellow fruits, and vegetables such as spinach, carrots, squash, sweet potatoes, peaches, cantaloupes. The usual daily complement of vitamin A [5,000 international units (IU) per day] will be supplied by your diet if you eat some portions of those fruits and vegetables and drink four glasses of vitamin A–fortified whole milk daily.

Too much vitamin A is dangerous. It is not soluble in water, and therefore excesses cannot be excreted in the urine. Instead, it accumulates in the liver and in other fatty tissues. It can cause liver failure, skin disease and loss of hair. What's more, it can produce similar and worse injuries in unborn children. It easily crosses the placenta and gets into the fetal tissues where it may cause defects in liver and bone growth. It has also been linked to a variety of birth defects. Vitamin A is not a harmless nutrient. When taken in large quantities (over a few thousand units per day) it becomes a dangerous drug, and your unborn child is a highly vulnerable target.

Vitamin D

A form of vitamin D can be made by the tissues of your body. It then sits under your skin waiting for you to activate it. How? By going out in the sunlight. Yes, sitting in the sun for an hour or two per day, if your climate permits, is a wholesome source of vitamin D. But most of us cannot get quite enough vitamin D this way, and very few of our usual foods contain it. Generally we get enough from fortified foods, particularly milk. If you eat adequate amounts of cheese, yogurt and milk that are fortified with vitamin D you should be able to get your full daily requirement of 400 IU recommended for the pregnant woman.

Small additional supplements are okay, but very large quantities of vitamin D can be dangerous. When taken in excess it produces calcium disturbances and can lead to loss of calcium from the bones and to deposition of calcium in places where it doesn't belong such as the heart and blood vessels. What's more, some individuals and particularly some unborn children are unusually sensitive to even small excesses of vitamin D. It has been well established that babies have been born with fatal or severely disabling calcification of their heart valve areas, caused by maternal vitamin D supplementation in a wide variety of dosages.[4,5]

Vitamin E

Relatively small quantities of vitamin E are required in pregnancy, as far as we know. All of the wondrous claims for large supplements of vitamin E have never been proven, although many attempts have been made. Once again, this doesn't close the door for all time. We may some day learn that the recommended amounts are insufficient, but for now, every indication tells us that you get enough if you adhere to the recommended daily food intakes. Hence, supplements are unnecessary. Whether or not too much vitamin E is dangerous isn't known, but it may be.

Vitamin K

Vitamin K plays an important role in normal blood-clotting. Without it, you would continue to bleed after you got cut. This vitamin apparently is needed in very small quantities, and the amount you get in your food is enough. Furthermore, you have another very large supply of the vitamin: the vast number of bacteria that live peacefully in your intestinal tract make vitamin K and pass it on to you. Vitamin K supplements are not needed. They may be harmful, particularly near the end of pregnancy, since too much vitamin K can give rise to a dangerous condition of neonatal jaundice (you recognize this as a yellow skin coloration).

Vitamin C

There is currently no support for the use of massive quantities of vitamin C. Sixty milligrams appears to be quite sufficient to keep mother healthy and produce healthy offspring, but because prepared food may have lost much of its active vitamin C, small supplements may be necessary. Or better, eat fresh fruits, every day, particularly fresh citrus fruits and juices. If you do this, you don't need supplements.

Might the current craze for massive vitamin C (500 to 2000 milligrams daily) harm the unborn child? No one knows. The potential adverse effects of the vitamin when taken in these amounts have not been studied. If you take that much vitamin C, you are taking a chance for yourself and your baby.

Folic Acid

This active little chemical, which is involved in scores of the body's chemical reactions, is found in many of our foods, including meats, liver, fresh fruits and many vegetables. The body's requirement for this vitamin is not great, but the need increases considerably during pregnancy. Some respected scientists feel that supplements of folic acid during pregnancy are required, while others disagree. The NRC says that women who choose their diets with care do not need supplemental folic acid, but your obstetrician may disagree with this. Since there is respectable opinion on both sides you may or may not take supplements, depending upon the quality of your diet and the recommendation of your personal physician.

Iron

There is also some debate about the need for supplemental iron in pregnancy. Iron, as you know, is mainly used to make healthy hemoglobin, the biochemical substance in our red blood cells that carries the oxygen from our lungs to the rest of our bodies—and in the pregnant woman, to her baby. One can calculate rather precisely the basic daily iron need during pregnancy, taking into account the amount needed by the growing fetus and the mother, and the amount lost through the mother's digestive tract. The NRC notes that the total additional iron requirements during pregnancy, when there is one fetus, are about 0.8 gms. Most diets, unless they include daily liver, do not provide that amount, so daily supplements of 30 mg of iron salts are usually recommended to make up the balance. Some people are concerned about the possible adverse consequences of these supplements, and a few animal studies have suggested possible harmful results. As far as we know, however, the recommended supplements are potentially more helpful than harmful.

Other Minerals and Salts

Besides iron, other major minerals and salts (with large quantities required) are calcium, magnesium, phosphorous, sodium and potassium. Minor ones (in quantity only, since they are certainly important) include iodine, copper, zinc, selenium, cobalt, chromium, manganese and probably others still to be discovered. Four glasses of milk per day, plus additional complements of dairy products and foods indicated in tables 2 and 3 provide the pregnant woman with what experts believe to be optimal daily requirements for all these minerals and salts. Presently there does not seem to be a need for supplementing any of them except, perhaps, calcium. However, if you diligently drink those four glasses of milk and eat cheese, and yogurt in between, calcium supplements won't be necessary.

An additional note: make sure you use iodized salt for all of your cooking and seasoning. The iodine concentration of supplemented salt is substantial and will obviate need for additional supplements.

Fiber

All of you who are concerned about good nutrition have heard a lot of talk lately about fibers. Fiber isn't truly a nutrient. It doesn't get into the body to be used for energy, chemical reactions or structure building. In fact, fiber's purpose in the diet is to remain in the intestinal tract, where it aids in digestion and elimination of wastes. Fiber helps keep you regular. It adds bulk to the stool and makes the passage of waste products much easier and smoother. This is very important in pregnancy, for constipation is one of the common problems that pregnant women suffer. It is far better to take care of this by increasing the fiber content of the diet than by taking potentially dangerous drugs, stool softeners or laxatives.

An important side effect of increasing dietary fiber is a greater natural vitamin and protein intake. You see, whole grains, less refined cereals, whole wheat and the new high-fiber breads are the best sources of dietary fiber. They should be eaten regularly instead of highly refined breads and cereals. They are also far better sources of vitamins and proteins, since, as mentioned earlier, refining and milling of flours and cereals destroy vitamins and proteins.

Summary

1. For the health of your children you must begin your program of good nutrition long before you actually become pregnant.
2. "Well-balanced" meals must be planned and selected with care.
3. In general, fresh fruits and vegetables and less processed breads and cereals offer better supplies of essential nutrients than do canned, bleached, milled, pasteurized and highly processed foods.
4. Look for fortified foods, particularly in milk and milk products.
5. Read the labels on boxes, cans, bottles, bread and cereal packages to check for vitamin, mineral, protein, fat, and carbohydrate contents.
6. Few supplements are required if you carefully plan your menu. Iron is the main exception. Since it generally isn't found in adequate quantity in most diets, small daily supplements are recommended. Some authorities also recommend supplemental calcium and folic acid.
7. Stay away from fad diets and massive vitamin and mineral supplements. Some may be dangerous.
8. Pregnancy is not a time for losing weight. A weight gain of 22 to 27 pounds is generally ideal.
9. For a comprehensive helpful guide to vitamin, protein, and caloric food values in every available food, refer to the guides listed in the reference section. You can find these at your local library or can purchase them from the publisher.

TABLE 1

Recommended Daily Dietary Allowances
for pregnant women. From the Food and Nutrition
Board, National Research Council, National
Academy of Sciences. Revised (1974).

Protein (gms)	70–80
Calories	2400
Vitamins	
Vitamin A (IU)	5000
Vitamin D (IU)	400
Vitamin E (IU)	15
Vitamin C (Ascorbic Acid) (mg)	60
Folic Acid (mg)	0.8
Niacin (mg)	15
Vitamin B_1 (Thiamine) (mg)	1.3
Vitamin B_2 (Riboflavin) (mg)	1.7
Vitamin B_6 (Pyridoxine) (mg)	2.5
Vitamin B_{12} (mg)	0.004
Minerals	
Calcium (mg)	1200
Phosphorous (mg)	1200
Iodine (mg)	.125
Iron (mg)	36
Magnesium (mg)	450
Zinc (mg)	20

TABLE 2

Recommended Daily Diet for the Pregnant Woman.

Milk and Milk Products

3 to 4 glasses of whole, fortified milk.
(Portion of cheese, yogurt, ice cream, or buttermilk
can be substituted for 1 glass)

Eggs

1 per day, may have 2 occasionally.

Fruits and Vegetables

Glass of juice (fresh if possible), or grapefruit half, or orange, or cantaloupe.

2 portions from the following list: green vegetables, tomatoes, potato (preferably with skin).

1 or 2 portions of yellow vegetable or fruit.

Meats and Meat Substitutes

2 servings of lean beef, chicken or other poultry or fish (2 to 4 ounces each). (A large serving of dried beans, nuts or peanut butter may occasionally be substituted for one of those portions of meat.)

3 to 4 ounces of liver should be eaten at least weekly, but no more than 3 times per week.

Breads and Cereals

4 portions daily of whole grain, preferably fortified breads and cereals. (One slice of bread equals one portion. ½ cup cereal equals one portion.)

Others

At least 2 tablespoons of butter, margarine or salad oil.

Cakes, candies, cookies to make up calories, but in limited quantities. Fresh fruits are far better desserts.

TABLE 3

Some Food Values in common foods. +- means
a trace. 1 fruit or vegetable refers to medium
size. For a more complete list the reader is referred
to the guides in the reference section.

	Calories	Protein gms	Calcium mg	Iron mg	VitA IU	Thiamine mg	Riboflavin mg	Niacin mg	VitC mg
Asparagus 4 spears	10	1	13	.4	540	.1	.1	.8	16
Broccoli 1 stalk	45	6	158	1.4	4500	.16	.36	1.4	163
Green beans 1 cup	30	2	63	.8	680	.09	.11	.6	15
Carrot, 1	20	1	18	.4	5500	.03	.03	.3	4
Potato, 1 baked	90	3	9	.7	+-	.1	.04	1.7	20
Tomato	40	2	24	.9	1640	.11	.07	1.3	30
Apple, 1	70	+-	8	.4	50	.04	.02	.1	3
Banana	100	1	10	.8	230	.06	.07	.8	12
Grapefruit ½ white	45	1	19	.5	10	.05	.02	.2	44
Grapefruit ½ pink	45	1	19	.5	540	.05	.02	.2	44
Orange juice	110	2	27	.5	500	.22	.07	1	124
Orange, 1	65	1	54	.5	260	.13	.05	.5	66
Peach, 1	35	1	9	.5	1320	.02	.05	1	7
Bread, whole w., 1 slice	65	3	24	.8	+-	.09	.03	.8	+-
Whole milk fortified, 1 cup	160	9	288	.1	350	.07	.41	.2	2
Cottage cheese 1 cup	260	33	230	.7	420	.07	.6	.2	0
American cheese, 1 oz	105	8	262	.3	320	+	.11	+	0

Yogurt 1 cup	125	8	294	.1	170	.1	.44	.2	2
Bacon 2 slices	90	5	2	.5	0	.08	.05	.8	0
Lean burger 3 oz	185	23	10	3	20	.08	.2	5	0
Lean steak 3 oz	220	24	10	3	20	.07	.19	4.8	0
Chicken, boiled 3 oz	115	20	8	1.4	80	.05	.16	7.4	0
Bluefish, baked 3 oz	135	22	25	.6	40	.09	.08	1.6	0
Peanut butter, 1 Tbsp.	95	4	9	.3	0	.02	.02	2.4	0
Liver, beef, 2 oz	130	15	6	5	30,280	.15	2.4	9.4	15
Egg, boiled, 1	80	6	27	1.1	590	.05	.15	+	0

Section Three
DRUGS

VII

What Are Drugs?

Drugs have accompanied man through history as inseparably as sickness and death. When early men succumbed to diseases, their priests and medicine men blamed vexed gods. They sought solutions first in incantations, sacrifices, prayers or rituals designed to appease or drive away unwanted spirits. Soon, herbs, berries, roots, potions and other concoctions became part of the healer's art. It was in these brews of the ancient Chinese, Egyptians and Sumerians that drug therapy was born.

The nostrums of these primitive medicine men seldom worked. In fact, they more often killed than cured. Strychnine, arsenic, mercury, extracts of mushrooms and hemlock and other powerful poisons were used by "healers" for thousands of years. Who knows how many hapless victims succumbed to these well-meant "cures"? But the value of the drug was rarely questioned, because disease, death and cures (if they ever occurred) were all seen as matters of faith. If the patient lived, the drug and the incantations were credited (though more often it was pure good luck or a mild illness that led to the favorable outcome).

For centuries these drugs went unchallenged. Finally, in the seventeenth and eighteenth centuries scientists and physicians began making some observations that sparked modern drug therapy. Astute healers observed that many of these ancient remedies could improve certain symptoms and cure some diseases. However, they had to be given in proper amounts. Too much could make the patient worse or even kill him. Some poisons of the past, such as strychnine, arsenic, extract of the foxglove plant (digitalis), the bark of the cinchona tree (quinine), were surprisingly useful remedies if they were used correctly. Amazingly, many of these ancient chemicals and extracts still play an important part in twentieth-century medicine. Frequently ancient healers were on the right track—they just didn't know how to control the drugs they had found.

For four thousand years, drugs were discovered by accident and prescribed by trial and error. Physicians of the eighteenth and nineteenth centuries began to control drug dosages, but only in the last 50 years has intelligent drug design really taken hold.

We have made major strides in drug planning, control and safety. We can design drugs that should, because we know their structures, combat certain illnesses. To a great extent, we can control the effectiveness of drugs. Those that work can be kept; those that don't, put aside. The most difficult problem has been controlling drug hazards. Some hazards can be eliminated, others identified and recognized, but many still escape detection. Unfortunately, almost every drug does things we don't want it to. These are known as side effects and complications. They may be quite serious for the one taking the drug and disastrous for that passive recipient, the unborn child.

How Drugs Work

Drugs work in many ways, and, although we still don't understand the details of all of them, we can fit most into a number of general categories.

Some drugs restore a normal body substance that has been lost by aging or disease. Insulin for the diabetic; thyroid hormone for one with an underactive thyroid gland; estrogens for the woman past menopause; cortisone for victims of Addison's disease (President Kennedy was one) are some examples.

Drugs may block or stimulate normal body functions

that have somehow gone awry. Common illnesses may be associated with a variety of imbalances which can be controlled this way. Antacids for ulcer sufferers; diuretics (water pills) and stronger medications for those with high blood pressure; decongestants to constrict blood vessels and counteract the stuffiness of colds and hay fever; anticoagulants (blood thinners) to prevent clotting after heart attacks or phlebitis, and digitalis to help power weakened heart muscles are among countless examples.

Drugs may block the signs and symptoms of an illness either by acting directly at the site of the problem or by short-circuiting it elsewhere—most often the brain. For example, aspirin may decrease the inflammation of swollen arthritic joints. It may also affect the perception of pain by working on pain pathways in the brain. Narcotics such as morphine also stop the brain from perceiving pain. Cortisone may abolish a rash due to poison ivy or a drug allergy. It somehow does this by directly interfering with the allergic reaction. Tranquilizers and sleeping pills act in the brain to alter nerve pathways—akin to throwing a circuit breaker or rerouting an electrical impulse.

Drugs may ward off invaders that attack us from the outside: antibiotics and antiseptics that fight infection are well known examples.

Drugs may battle internal derangements that threaten our lives: anticancer drugs are potent warriors against malignant growths.

Finally, certain drugs may help marshal the body's own defenses against external assaults. Vaccines against polio, diphtheria, whooping cough, tetanus, measles and many others help organize our immune systems to a state of readiness should these diseases threaten. You and your children have all been given drugs like these.

Drug Risks

With this variety of drugs, disease and discomfort are better controlled than ever before. But the adage,

"You don't get something for nothing," might have been written about drugs, for none of them is devoid of risk.

The possible dangers fall into two general types. They may be extensions of the intended action of the drug—in a sense, "too much of a good thing." Or they may be totally new threats, often at a site far removed from the intended target of the drug. These distant effects may be due to direct toxicity of the drug or they may be due to allergic reactions, the body's way of rejecting and fighting an unwanted intruder.

The unborn child, because he is so small and his organs so immature, is frighteningly sensitive to those same toxic effects to which you are sensitive. Unwanted excesses of the drug's action and threats to innocent organs are even more ominous for him. In addition, he is menaced by other unique dangers.

For one thing, the process of normal body and organ development may be thrown hopelessly out of kilter, giving rise to a vast variety of birth defects. Many of these are gross malformations. Others may be considerably harder to detect, such as subtle alterations in mental and physical development.

Secondly, the newborn infant's brain, unlike the adult's, is exquisitely sensitive to drug-induced imbalances in a blood waste called bilirubin. Most babies are born with some degree of jaundice—they appear yellow. The yellow color comes from this chemical waste product, bilirubin, which is normally handled by the liver and passed out through the bile into the feces. Babies are yellow, or jaundiced, because their immature livers don't get rid of the bilirubin efficiently.

What does this have to do with drugs? A great deal. Many drugs can markedly increase the normal amount of neonatal jaundice by either acting on the liver directly and impairing its handling of the bilirubin, or by separating the bilirubin from certain blood proteins to which it is normally bound. The outcome can be very serious, for the newborn can tolerate some jaundice, but not too much. Excessive jaundice can lead to an illness known as kernicterus which produces permanent and devastating brain malfunction.

This complication can be caused by a number of drugs. It only occurs when the drug is taken near delivery, since the newborn infant, not the fetus, is the one who is susceptible. Those drugs that produce neonatal jaundice, therefore, differ from those that produce congenital deformities (keeping in mind that some may do both), since congenital deformities generally arise from assaults during the first trimester and the early part of the second trimester, when organ development is most active.

Thus, some drugs may be dangerous near the end of the pregnancy and harmless at the beginning. Others may be disastrous early but benign later. Still others, like aspirin which apparently causes congenital defects as well as neonatal problems, are risky throughout. Later, we will explore times and types of hazards that go with specific drugs in more detail. For now, let us consider a few to illustrate the general classes of drug risks.

Too Much of the Intended Response

Insulin

If you are diabetic you may have to take insulin. The survival of both you and your baby may depend upon it. However, if you do need insulin, the dosage must be carefully monitored. Required amounts often change drastically during pregnancy. Insulin lowers the blood sugar concentration. The more you take, the lower your blood sugar level goes. If it goes too low, your cells can't work properly and you lose consciousness. Your unborn child depends on you for his sugar. As yours falls, his falls. Too much of the necessary drug insulin may rob the growing child of vital sugar and permanently injure growing parts or kill him before birth.

Antithyroid Medication

If the fact that you are severely hyperthyroid has been confirmed by proper testing, you may have to take special medication to reduce your thyroid activity, even though you are pregnant. The problem: the drug may enter the growing child and affect the growth and development of his immature thyroid gland. He may thus be born with low thyroid function, a condition commonly known as cretinism, and may need thyroid replacement medication to function properly. Thus, for you, an adult, a dosage of antithyroid medication is just right. For your unborn child, minute in size, that dosage can be overwhelming.

Anticoagulants (blood thinners)

Occasionally pregnant women develop problems with blood clots in their legs or the very serious condition of clots in their lungs. At times anticoagulant medications are mandatory. Too much causes an exaggeration of the intended blood-thinning effect and may lead to bleeding. The fetus is particularly susceptible. Coumarin, the most common oral anticoagulant, crosses the placenta and gets into the baby. Fetal injuries due to bleeding before or during birth have occurred. Some have been extremely serious and have led to death or to lifelong brain injuries. Fortunately, modern pharmacology has brought us an effective solution. Another anticoagulant, heparin does not cross the placenta and will not cause fetal bleeding. It is a bit harder to use, since it can't be taken orally but must be injected. However, the added safety for the baby is worth it, and most obstetricians now use heparin rather than coumarin if anticoagulation is mandatory.

Diuretics (water pills)

If you're like most women, you've probably noted some swelling of your ankles, particularly around period time or during pregnancy. Many of you have taken diuretics at some time—all too often, when you were pregnant.

Diuretics, used to treat high blood pressure and fluid retention, help the kidneys to excrete salt and water. Scientists now feel that the extra fluid that causes your ankle swelling is probably important to a normal pregnancy. Loss of too much salt and water may hamper fetal growth.

This makes good sense, since it is hard to imagine that something as common as ankle swelling in pregnancy could be abnormal. Nature doesn't work that way. If water accumulation is massive and dangerous, it must be treated. Otherwise, diuretics should not be routinely used in pregnancy. The unborn child may be the unfortunate victim of too much of an intended drug response: in this case, water and salt elimination.

Effects on Other Organs

Many drugs produce undesired side effects and complications at sites far removed from the planned target. Here we mention just a few that may be important to the growing fetus.

Antibiotics

Certain potent bacteria-fighters such as streptomycin, kanamycin, gentamicin and others may be life-saving to the individual threatened by deadly bacteria. They may also take their own toll, particularly on two organs, far apart and seemingly quite different from one another: the inner ears and the kidneys. The hearing and balance mechanisms located in the inner ear may be wiped out by any of those drugs, which produce dizziness, deafness or both.

The kidneys are equally sensitive and can be destroyed by them.

The unborn child is not immune. In fact, he is probably more sensitive than his mother who is taking the drugs. Thus, these drugs must be used with great caution by the pregnant woman, and only if absolutely necessary. If not, the baby may die of kidney failure or may be born to a life of total deafness.

Quinine

This is a drug which is used to combat malaria, but is more familiar to you in a summer drink—gin and tonic. The tonic is flavored with quinine and quinine can injure the sight mechanism and even produce blindness by damaging the retina—the back of the eye where images are perceived. Some people are more sensitive than others to this adverse effect. Does the usual gin and tonic produce this effect? Probably not, because the concentration of quinine is too low. But it may not be too low for the more vulnerable fetus. A simple social drink, one which you don't even consider a drug, may be dangerous to your growing child.

Narcotics

Narcotics are addicting. This dependency, an unwanted side effect of these useful pain relievers, is probably due to a variety of body changes, particularly in the brain. Unfortunately, newborns of addicted mothers enter the world addicted. Their bodies have suffered the same changes as their mothers' at the most vulnerable time in their lives. They require highly skilled medical care to break the habit and save their lives. They are the pathetic victims of a drug complication.

Narcotics, Barbiturates, Tranquilizers

These sedatives and pain relievers are frequently given during labor and delivery to comfort the mother. Their major side effect is depression of respiration. This can be a problem for the mother herself if too much of these drugs is given, and even more so for the newborn. They readily cross the placenta, and reasonable doses for his mother may be much too much for him. Babies whose mothers are given these drugs shortly before delivery must be watched very carefully. They may stop breathing altogether or just enough to cause brain damage. They may require artificial respiration until they can rid their bodies of these depressant drugs and breathe on their own.

Aspirin

Aspirin, it is now known, can cause bleeding. This unwanted side effect may endanger the fetus, particularly at birth. Many newborns whose mothers took aspirin near delivery time have suffered serious bleeding —victims of a seemingly harmless drug.

Mood-altering Drugs

There is a constellation of possible harmful drug actions which is unexplored, rarely considered, but frightening in its implications. How does the fetus respond to the mind-altering effects of the sleeping pills, stimulants (coffee included), and tranquilizers, all downed indiscriminately by many women today? These drugs alter adult perceptions, emotions and physical and mental activity. The vast majority easily invade the baby's tissues. In the past, few considered the possibility that the fetus might experience any emotional or mental life. In fact, he probably does, although exactly what form this takes remains a secret. Certainly the child hears and responds to noises. He feels his environment, sucks his thumb and moves about. He may even see. His brain, though not fully developed, has many adult characteristics long before birth. He may not think the way we do, but brain cells are there. They carry some sort of primitive messages, and they are undoubtedly susceptible to drug influences. Stimulants and depressants which alter perception, mood and consciousness must have some effect on the unborn child. How dangerous the effect, and how or when it may show up after birth, we don't yet know.

Teratogenesis

Teratogenesis (producing birth defects) is the best-known and the most dread of all adverse drug effects. A number of drugs have now been identified as clear culprits. Many, probably the vast majority, have not. We traced in Chapter 3 the exquisitely balanced process of fetal growth and development. It's not hard to imagine that a foreign chemical might be taken up by the growing tissues and throw the process into disarray. Drugs are foreign chemicals. They don't belong in the environment of the growing fetus. A certain number of them will play havoc with the intricate events of fetal development.

Most teratogens remain unknown. They are mysterious but often devastating assailants of our unborn children. They carefully guard their secrets, almost mockingly beckoning us to find them out. Why they often win this game of hide-and-seek is the topic of the next chapter.

VIII

Drug Safety—A Myth?

Tina Miller gazed sadly into the crib, her mind bursting with thoughts of the future. There her two-week-old daughter lay sleeping. Angelic, beautiful, a perfect baby, you would surely say. But the blanket tucked snugly under the infant's chin hid a tragic story; Alissa had no arms. Instead, five fingers and a small wrist dangled pathetically from each of her shoulders.

"How could this have happened?" wailed Tina. "Why our child?"

This was the crushing reality for thousands of families in the 1960s; victims of the drug thalidomide. For the parents of these children, the adjustments, the pressures, the guilt, were agonizing. For the children, daily activities, simple for normal youngsters, were insurmountable tasks.

"Those years are over," you think. "This is a new era of fail-safe medicines and harmless drugs. Our Food and Drug Administration (FDA) will see to it that a new thalidomide story will never unfold."

Wishful thinking and, unfortunately, untrue. Drug testing is never absolutely reliable. Even if the FDA, the pharmaceutical companies and practicing physicians do their best (and many doubt that they do), dangerous drugs slip by. As we move along in the chapter you will begin to understand why. For now, accept the premise that if you are pregnant no drug can be assumed harmless. The FDA, your doctor and the pharmaceutical companies may be on your side, but you're the one who must take final responsibility. After all, it's your baby.

Begin with a fresh approach to drugs. Forget the propaganda of TV advertising: the giant-size nose with the dribbles, the head with the hammer pounding away inside, the stomach burning up with "excess" acid, the long-faced, middle-aged woman with a touch of "irregularity." Don't run to the medicine chest or the druggist's shelf every time you have the "blahs," "simple nervous tension," "acid stomach," "sinus trouble," or that "ache-all-over feeling."

Before you pick up a pill, capsule, tablet or a spoonful of liquid medicine, ask yourself, "Is it worth taking the chance?" Chance? Yes, taking any drug means taking a chance. This may require a total about-face in your thinking, but it is true. No drug—not aspirin, penicillin, antacids, cold remedies, sinus medicines, diuretics (water pills), pills for morning sickness or any other, whether they come from your druggist's display case or by prescription—can be taken with absolute confidence that it won't harm your growing child.

Equally important, this about-face in your thoughts and deeds must begin well before you find out that you're pregnant. Recall how the baby grows: most of the organs are well under way to full formation before you even suspect that you are pregnant. Many drugs, particularly the ones that destroy or deform the fetus, do their harm during those critical starting weeks. So it won't do to clean those pills out of the medicine chest when the pregnancy test comes back positive. By then it is too late. Good drug habits, which more often than not means no drugs at all, must become a way of life from the moment that pregnancy —accidental or planned—becomes a possibility.

Does this mean that anything you may take will surely—or even likely—injure your unborn child? You may be thinking, "I took aspirin, water pills and medicine for morning sickness the last time I was pregnant, and my child is as healthy as can be. And my girlfriend was nervous, so she was given tranquilizers and sleeping pills during pregnancy. Everything came out just fine." There's no argument—more often than not, you'll get away with taking drugs. The incidence of visible injuries caused by most (but not all) drugs is still quite low. However, your child runs a far greater risk of bearing a lifelong, possibly disastrous, scar if you expose him to drugs than if you carefully shelter him.

Thank goodness every drug taken doesn't lead to a birth injury. Studies in this country have come up with alarming figures about drug use in pregnancy. As many as 90% of pregnant women take some drugs during pregnancy; an average of 4.5 drugs, most self-prescribed, are used; as many as 4% of pregnant women take 10 or more different drugs.[1-3]

Studies also show that the incidence of birth defects is rising in this country and that America, with all of its modern medical marvels, ranks only sixteenth among Western countries at keeping its newborns alive.[4] How much of this rise in birth defects and high perinatal mortality is due to drugs used in pregnancy, we don't know. Many believe, however, that our cultural mania for drugs-for-every-ill may be a major contributor.[1-3,5-6]

Yes, you might take a drug with no ill effect. The odds are still in your and your child's favor—but it is a gamble, and the stake is the health and welfare of your baby.

The manufacturer's warning that physicians receive with all drug packages and the cautions in the "Physician's Desk Reference" (the common medical guide to drugs) range from the mild admonition: "The safety of (this drug) . . . during pregnancy and lactation has not been established. It should not be used in women of childbearing potential unless the expected benefits outweigh the possible hazards;" to stronger embargoes: ". . . can be teratogenic (producing fetal abnormalities, sic) or, cause fetal resorption in experimental animals. It should not be used in pregnancy, particularly early pregnancy, unless in the judgment of the physician, the potential benefits outweigh the possible risks."

The element of risk/benefit that we discussed earlier

is always mentioned, as well it should be, for there are times when drug therapy is mandatory.

Take note of this caveat, recently issued by the Committee on Drugs of the American Academy of Pediatrics: "There is no drug, whether over-the-counter remedy or prescription drug, which, when taken by or administered to a childbearing woman, has been proven safe for the unborn child."[7]

Why can't we ensure the safety of drugs? Why can't our FDA and the pharmaceutical companies see to it that every marketed drug is free from hazard? The answers are many. In the first place, drugs are chemicals, designed to serve a purpose, but they are foreign to the body. Every one of them, from aspirin to penicillin, can produce side effects and complications. Though these can be minimized, they can never be eliminated entirely.

When it comes to a drug's adverse effects on the growing child, we are faced with a whole new complex of potential complications, many of which can never be fully tested. The thalidomide story is a fascinating example of how a drug so harmful to the growing fetus was mass-marketed and only later exposed. Behind the scenes of this story is a striking lesson that shows why other harmful drugs may never be weeded out.

Thalidomide was first introduced in Germany in the late 1950s. To the credit of our FDA it was never approved for use in this country. American women who took it generally obtained it during travels in Germany. The drug was tested in animals. It was found to be safe. We learned too late that animals are far less susceptible to the mutilating effects of thalidomide. Man is 60 times more sensitive than mice, 100 times more sensitive than rats, 200 times more than dogs and 700 times more than hamsters.[8,9] Consequently, the potential dangers to man were never uncovered in animal tests. Man turned out to be the "guinea pig."

The drug was a useful and effective sedative. Alas, it was shortly discovered that it brought relief from morning sickness. Pregnant women soon became the major users, and this drug, given to help them through their pregnancies, was on its way to becoming the scourge of modern medicine.

In late 1961, a clever German pediatrician made an ominous observation: a recent astounding increase in the rate of phocomelia (the characteristic arm and leg abnormalities produced by thalidomide).[10] What's more, that pediatrician noted that all of the cases of phocomelia shared a common feature—each of the mothers had taken thalidomide. The association was quickly confirmed; the drug stopped, but for 10,000 babies it was too late. They bore, forever, the deforming scars of this mutilating drug.[11-13]

The thalidomide tragedy points out why fetal immunity to drugs can never be ensured. For one thing, animal testing is rarely ironclad. Thalidomide was tested in pregnant animals, but they were less susceptible to its effects than human beings. Next, unlike the vast majority of drug risks, the hazards of thalidomide were uncovered early. Prompt detection occurred for three reasons, rather unique to this drug: first, it was given to a large number of pregnant women at precisely the time when the fetuses were most vulnerable; second, the injuries were bizarre and previously quite uncommon; third, the incidence of birth defects in exposed fetuses was probably high.

Thalidomide left obvious clues that guided scientists to its discovery. Other drugs may injure the growing child, but most hide their secrets far better than thalidomide. If they are identified at all, it may only be after causing many years of heartache.[14]

"Why can't modern science and our government agencies do a better job?" you may be wondering.

For one thing, no organization is directly charged with monitoring birth defects. This means that if you, your neighbor, a friend or a relative has a deformed child, no one may ever ask the right questions: "What drugs did you take? What household products did you use? Did you have any illnesses? Did you work in a plant or factory that perhaps exposed you to noxious fumes?"

If the pediatrician caring for the child happens to be

particularly astute or concerned he might probe into your history during those nine months. He might even report any positive answers, particularly about drugs, to the FDA. However, the system is entirely voluntary and haphazard. Thousands of deformed children never become part of these essential surveys. Thus potential hazards may continue unrecognized and unchallenged.

What happens to those reports that are submitted to the FDA? They are filed and cross-referenced, and when enough reports point to a particular drug, an investigation may follow. To prove that a drug caused the birth defect—that it wasn't merely an innocent bystander—is much harder than it may seem. An example may help show why. Your child was born with a heart defect. You took a cold preparation for four days during your third month of pregnancy. Did the medication produce the defect? Was it the cold itself, another illness, your improper diet, the insecticides that you sprayed in the garden, or just a freak of nature? If two hundred more identical birth defects are reported to the FDA and all of the mothers took the same drug that you did, the kernel of suspicion may begin to grow. The culprit may eventually be identified.

Thalidomide roared thunderously into view. It was used by thousands of pregnant women and left characteristic mutilation in its wake. By comparison, many other drugs are like cat burglars, striking quietly, leaving no clues. Potentially dangerous drugs may be used only occasionally by pregnant women, unlike thalidomide, which was used almost exclusively during pregnancy. Thus, its threat to the growing fetus, may never be recognized, since unborn children would be so rarely exposed.

Or a drug may be used commonly, but only rarely produce any harm. Aspirin is an example. How difficult it is to pinpoint such a culprit! When asked if she took any drugs (if anyone bothers to ask), the mother of a damaged child might not even remember to mention aspirin, so common is it to everyday life. If she did note the few aspirin tablets that she took, the thousands of normal pregnancies among mothers who ingested aspirin would give statisticians fits. They would find it most difficult to prove that aspirin was the cause. Would you for a moment consider aspirin the likely cause of your child's injury? Neither did the FDA, until recently. (See next chapter.)

Finally, a drug may produce a birth defect which is relatively common—one which has many possible causes and frequently occurs in women who did not take any drug at all. Cleft lip is a common developmental abnormality. A large number of children are born with this defect. Careful investigation has told us that it often is not related to any drug history. If a mother gives birth to a child with this deformity, and she had taken a certain drug, how do we know whether or not the drug played a role? The answer: when the injury produced is a common one we often can't be sure that a drug was responsible. Precisely the opposite was true of thalidomide. It produced an injury which was so unusual that the link to the drug was uncovered quite early.

Recently another drug disaster has cropped up which poignantly illustrates the problems of assuring drug safety in pregnancy. By now you have probably heard of the drug DES (diethylstilbestrol). The papers and magazines have literally exploded with the strange and frightening tale of this drug.

DES is closely related to the normal female hormone estrogen. It was used extensively throughout the 1950s and 1960s to treat problems of pregnancy including bleeding, cramps, threatened miscarriages and prevention of miscarriages in women who had had a number previously.[15,16] By all accounts, by all the usual measures of drug testing, it was safe. Because many obstetricians believed that it was both safe and effective and because the problems for which it was recommended were quite common, many pregnant women were given DES—perhaps as many as two million.

But in 1971, a group of obstetricians from Harvard Medical School made a startling observation that rocked both medical and public communities. An unusual type of vaginal cancer was identified in six young women between 14 and 22 years old.[17] What's more they all shared a second common feature: each of them had been exposed to DES while they were still inside their mothers. Other reports followed rapidly and the association was confirmed.[18-20] Gynecologists around the world were soon convinced that DES could cause the belated appearance of genital tract cancers in young women. The latent period was remarkable —usually 15 years or more. This was the first time in the history of pharmacology that such a delayed effect on the exposed fetus had ever been identified.

Before long, other conditions of the female reproductive tract were linked to this exposure to DES in the distant past.[21-23] Fortunately, these others are all benign, but no one is quite sure whether they may lead to cancerous changes. To date, only 280 cancers have been reported out of an estimated 500,000 to 1,000,-000 exposed women.[24] Thousands of benign abnormalities have been uncovered, and physicians everywhere share the public's hope that the toll of malignancies doesn't escalate.

How dramatically this DES story illustrates our message. Here we have an effect, unpredictable by usual testing, a shock to gynecologists, potentially catastrophic for scores of young women. The victims were women exposed 15 or more years ago, before they were even born. Their mothers are profoundly remorseful, blaming themselves for something over which neither they, their physicians, the FDA, nor the pharmaceutical companies had any control at the time.

Drugs were the hope of modern medicine in the 1950s, but pregnant women were not placed in a special class. Now, one hopes, we have ascended to a new level of sophistication, though the frightening drug-use statistics quoted earlier make us wonder. Pregnant women are unique. They carry another vulnerable person. If the DES disaster hasn't taught us a lesson, such a tragedy is bound to happen again.

IX

Common Drugs in
Your Medicine Cabinet

Americans have a passion for drugs. They're the easy answers to all of our problems, real and imagined. Spurred on by millions of dollars worth of electronic and printed advertising, we've found a remedy for every twinge of distress. Heartburn, gas, constipation, diarrhea, headache, backache, muscle aches, sinus headaches, allergy, anxiety, simple nervous tension, insomnia—all are conditions that bring to mind Madison Avenue jingles. The subjects of many of those jingles are prominently displayed in most medicine chests.

Pills and potions are ingrained in our culture—a part of our daily lives. Think for a moment: don't you regard aspirin as a "simple" pain reliever and not as a drug with dangers and side effects? It's easy to understand how this feeling of complacency about drugs persists during pregnancy. You wouldn't dream that simple aspirin might cause birth defects or lead to serious problems such as bleeding in the newborn. Well, as noted earlier, it can.

Let's briefly explore the world of some of those common inhabitants of our medicine cabinets. While all too often these may include prescription drugs such as diuretics, tranquilizers and antinausea, antivomiting and sleeping medications, we'll reserve the discussion of those until later. For now, let's consider the over-the-counter remedies—the ones you can buy without a physician's prescription.

Aspirin (Acetylsalicylic Acid)

If your pain or headache is so mild that aspirin will help, forget it. Try a warm towel on your forehead, a warm glass of milk or a nap. They're much better and far safer. If you are one of the comparatively few individuals with a serious disease such as rheumatoid arthritis that requires aspirin therapy, you have no choice. For you, the risk is necessary. For most of you who take the drug for simple problems, it isn't.

But is there really a risk from aspirin? What damage can aspirin do?

The three major fetal injuries that have been linked to aspirin are: death, congenital deformities, and bleeding of the newborn.[1-10]

A number of studies have found a higher incidence of fetal death when mothers frequently took aspirin, usually for minor problems and almost always self-prescribed. One, a recent Australian study, showed an alarming increase in both stillborn rate and perinatal death when mothers took aspirin constantly during pregnancy.[9,10] And even for those who took it only sporadically, the incidence of fetal and newborn disasters was higher. Other studies have reached similar conclusions. It is relatively certain that aspirin, particularly when taken frequently, but probably when used occasionally as well, does jeopardize the fetus and make him less likely to survive the full pregnancy.

Rats, mice, rabbits and monkeys, exposed to aspirin before birth, have repeatedly merged with a host of birth defects. Cleft palate, cleft lip, brain abnormalities, shriveled limbs, growth retardation, eye deformities, digestive tract malformations are some of the many aftermaths of aspirin exposure.[11-15] The relationship of these animals' experiences to human beings is uncertain. Skeptics remind us that the dosage employed generally exceeded considerably the human dosages (on a relative per-weight basis). True, but let's not forget that human and animal sensitivities to drugs may vary profoundly. The thalidomide story recalls a sad example, for experimental animals were far less sensitive to the drug than human beings. Therefore the animal studies were always negative even though the dosages greatly exceeded human levels.

What if the same were true for aspirin? What if human beings were more sensitive than experimental animals? Then those animal dosages that may seem too high to concern us could actually pose a serious threat. The only safe conclusion is that abnormalities in test animals, even if the dosages are high, should raise a red flag of caution. We may be wrong, but we're sure to be safe if we put some stock in those positive studies.

Recently some human studies have supported these animal findings. Mental retardation, limb abnormalities and other developmental defects may occur more frequently in offspring of regular aspirin users. Moreover, this risk may be enhanced by today's processed and preserved food world. Benzoic acid, a common food preservative, is structurally related to aspirin. Teratogenic effects of aspirin, at least in experimental animals, are apparently augmented by feeding benzoic acid.[16] The term synergism is used to describe this enhanced effect of one chemical by another. Thus, it is possible, that even usual or small dosages of aspirin may become increasingly dangerous as this food additive is more widely used. Although these animal and human studies are still being questioned and examined, we are left with only one safe logical conclusion. A drug like aspirin—usually unessential—isn't worth taking any chances at all.

The arguments about teratogenic effects of aspirin in humans remain unsettled, but other very serious fetal complications are now widely accepted. Aspirin, particularly when taken too near delivery time, poses a real danger. It readily crosses the placenta and gets into the baby's circulation. We have learned in recent years that aspirin has significant anticlotting effects, and the baby is particularly sensitive. This means that babies born shortly after their mothers take aspirin are prone to developing bleeding problems at delivery or soon thereafter. Remember, birth is traumatic. The baby gets pushed and banged around trying to get out. If he has a tendency to bleed, he can have trouble, ranging from simple bruises under the skin to massive bleeding under the skull that may squeeze his brain and kill him. Children have died as a result of aspirin-related perinatal bleeding.

Now that you know that you shouldn't take aspirin while you are pregnant you should know which drugs contain it. The list is so long it could fill the next 10 pages, so let me give you some general classes of aspirin-containing drugs and then implore you to do one thing: read the label! Aspirin is formally known as acetylsalicylic acid or acetylsalicylate and it will probably be listed that way. You may also see the ingredients salicylate or salicylamide which are very closely related and should be avoided.

In addition to the obvious, pills that say aspirin on the bottle, almost all the other over-the-counter pain relievers are basically aspirin. This includes all of the best-known brand names like Excedrin, Alka-Seltzer, Anacin, and Bufferin. Many of the sinus medicines contain aspirin. Many cold remedies contain aspirin. Some sedatives and sleeping medications contain it. Dristan, Sine Off, Sine-Aid, 4-Way Cold Tablets, Doans Pills, Sominex, are others that contain aspirin or related compounds. Probably 80 percent of the drugs that you habitually pick up without a prescription contain aspirin. So, please . . . read the label!

Chloroform

You may not realize that you have had chloroform on your medicine shelf—and by now it may be gone. The FDA has recently proposed a ban on chloroform in pharmaceutical products, and we can hope the ban will hold up without a successful challenge. Chloroform, you see, was recently found to be cancer-producing in rats and mice, and it also has produced birth defects in experimental animals. Believe it or not, over 2,000 products from cough remedies to toothpastes contained chloroform as of June 1976. This should now be past history, but if chloroform products are still being made, avoid them. You can find out which they are by sending for a special booklet put out by the FDA. Any drug that causes cancer, whether remotely suspected or proven like chloroform, should be avoided if at all possible. Cancer producers are likely to also be teratogenic.

Antacids

Tums, Rolaids, Maalox, Gelusil, Digel, Alka-Seltzer, and Pepto Bismol are household names, consumed by the ton for upset stomachs. But these tablets and liquids that we so nonchalantly chew or swallow may not be as harmless as they seem. The data isn't strong, but at least one study suggested a higher rate of birth defects in offspring of mothers taking these drugs.[4] Sometimes the heartburn of pregnancy can be pretty miserable, but the best advice is to be cautious. You might take small doses of antacids occasionally if you are extremely uncomfortable, but don't make it a regular habit.

Tranquilizers,
Sleeping Medications

Most over-the-counter drugs to combat insomnia and nervous tension have as their active ingredients antihistamines: most often methapyrilene or pyrilamine; sometimes both. Sominex, Nytol, Sleep-Eze, Compoz, to name a few of the more common brands, are among them. Moreover, some contain aspirin. We know very little about the effects of these antihistamines on the fetus. The only information is that a couple of studies have produced congenital deformities in animals with pyrilamine.[17,18] The best policy, since these drugs are usually not essential, is to put them aside while you are pregnant.

Cough Remedies

Some of the over-the-counter cough remedies contain a variety of extraneous decongestants and other drugs, in addition to the active ingredient. Unless your cough is quite severe, you shouldn't take anything. If it is violent and relentless, it might itself be undesirable for the baby. Have your physician give you a single-ingredient cough suppressant: either dextromethorphan, or, even better, a low dosage of codeine.

Sinus Medications, Cold Remedies, Other Pain Medications

As noted earlier, many sinus medicines and cold remedies contain aspirin, so don't take them unless absolutely necessary. They also contain a variety of antihistamines and decongestants, most of which aren't known to be deleterious but haven't been well studied. Thus, if you take a sinus medication, you take a chance.

The other major over-the-counter pain medication, besides aspirin, is acetaminophen, commonly sold as Tylenol or Datril. We have no idea about the effect of this drug on the fetus, because few if any studies have been done. It, too, carries the aura of uncertainty, and since it is a mild medication which can generally be done without, try to avoid it.

Antihistamines Used for Motion Sickness

After the thalidomide incident many studies were carried out on motion-sickness medications which are also frequently used for morning sickness. Be aware of their chemical names: cyclizine, meclizine, diphenhydramine, promethazine, pyrilamine, although some may be sold under specific brand names, including Bonine, Benadryl, Phenergan and Antivert. Today some of these are available by prescription only, and others are presently sold over the counter. Most of these drugs have been implicated in the genesis of various deformities in experimental animals.[19-23] Some human studies are purported to identify similar hazards, but these were not comprehensive or well performed.[24,25]

Because these drugs are used extensively to treat morning sickness, the FDA gathered data from a large group of well-designed human studies. The results showed no increase in fetal deformities when these drugs were administered.[26-28]

Severe vomiting associated with pregnancy may necessitate some drug treatment, but since the merits and drawbacks of these drugs have not been fully resolved, and since many animal studies are alarming, use these drugs with care. Don't buy them on your own. Consult your physician and take them only if you can't get along without them.

Summary

1. Avoid most over-the-counter medications during pregnancy. The minor symptoms for which they are designed—heartburn, headache, sinus trouble, allergies, sleeplessness, colds, minor cough, etc.—are annoying, but they are rarely sufficiently troublesome to warrant any risk, however remote, to your unborn child.
2. Aspirin is dangerous. Avoid it. If you have a serious problem that requires aspirin therapy, discuss it with your physician. If your health or your baby's health may be jeopardized if you don't take this drug, you may have no choice.
3. Read labels on all medications. Aspirin is often there.
4. Don't self-medicate while you are pregnant. If symptoms are severe, call your doctor.

X

Drugs for Common Complaints of Pregnancy

Pregnancy is usually a happy time. You look forward with anticipation to the birth of your new child. Your underlying mood is joyful, but that doesn't mean that every moment is fun and games. Pregnancy can bring loads of nagging physical annoyances. Aches, pains, tiredness, nausea, vomiting, indigestion and swollen ankles may be the price for that "bundle of joy."

When these irritating problems arise, the natural desire is to want to get rid of them. "I'll take something," may be your first thought. You may run to the drugstore (or send your husband), rummage through those dusty bottles in the medicine chest, or phone your doctor for a prescription. By now we've harped on this enough for you to appreciate why a quick cure for every ill is a bad idea when you're pregnant.

Sometimes it may even be dangerous to call your doctor. Does that sound like blasphemy? Let us explain: we don't dislike doctors—we are doctors ourselves. When you are sick a doctor is "just what the doctor ordered." If you have a serious or unusual problem or even a question, by all means, call your doctor. The welfare of both you and your baby may depend upon it.

If, however, you call your physician for every ache and pain that are part of all pregnancies, you may find yourself taking a drug you don't really need. This is particularly likely to happen if you give your doctor the impression that you want to take something. You see, your physician is under some pressure to give you drugs. You want relief; he wants to please you. He may decide that your happiness and good will are worth taking some chance—"probably small, after all" —for your unborn child. Or, if you nag him enough, he may just want to get you off his back.

Surely you would agree that a drug ordered merely to control mild ills, to stop your complaining, or to cut down the doctor's phone calls, is a poor reason to expose your unborn child to even the smallest risk. The only justification for a drug is to treat a serious illness that threatens you or your child, or to counteract severe symptoms or discomfort that are truly a major problem for you. The vast majority of pregnancy complaints, although irritating, are harmless. Occasional morning sickness, mild ankle swelling, a few aches and pains can be bothersome, but they'll pass and you and your baby will be no worse off for them. For the most part, however, the drugs you take serve one purpose and one purpose only: to make you feel better. This places the responsibility squarely on your shoulders, not on your doctor's. You have to decide whether you are bothered so badly that you are willing to expose your unborn child to drugs which may or may not be harmful. You are the only one who truly knows how bad you feel and how urgently you need relief.

Now let us explore some of the problems you might face during your pregnancy, and the drugs most often used to control them. Morning sickness, heartburn, headaches, abdominal pains, constipation, hemorrhoids, and swollen ankles from fluid retention are a few of the common ailments that annoy most pregnant women.

Morning Sickness

Nausea and vomiting, a problem of most pregnancies, is usually worse during the first trimester, then gradually tapers off. Most often the symptoms occur in the morning, hence the familiar name, but this annoying stomach upset can strike at any time of the day. Try to control your symptoms with dietary changes, rather than with drugs. Smaller, more frequent meals; blander, easier-to-digest foods will often make you comfortable enough to do without drugs. Sometimes eating will actually decrease your nausea.

Occasionally nausea and vomiting can be incapacitating. If your morning sickness is that bad and changes in diet haven't helped, you may have no choice but to take some medication. Severe, out-of-control vomiting can make you miserable, impair your food intake and nutrition, and threaten your baby's welfare.

The drugs that are commonly used to control morning sickness include a variety of antihistamines and tranquilizers. After the thalidomide disaster, most of these drugs were tested extensively to see whether or not they posed any threat to the unborn child. As we noted in the last chapter, the answers are inconclusive. Most of them can produce birth deformities in laboratory animals. A few human studies also purported to show a higher incidence of birth defects in children exposed to these drugs, others have not (see refs. Chapter 9). Many, many women have taken these drugs with no adverse consequences; thus, if they are harmful, the incidence is probably relatively low. They're clearly not as dangeous as thalidomide. Don't let anyone tell you, however, that "they are perfectly safe." No one knows that, and we doubt that they are.

For the moment there is no known difference in risk for any of the commonly used drugs. Some of their family names include meclizine, cyclizine, dimenhydrinate, and doxylamine. These are sold under a variety of brand names. If you are suffering badly from morning sickness, if you are vomiting all or most of your meals, go ahead and accept a prescription from your doctor. Remember, however, only you know how bad your symptoms are—your doctor only knows what you tell him. Also, take them as seldom as possible— only when symptoms are severe—and stop them as soon as you can.

Indigestion, Gas
and Heartburn

Very few of you will go through an entire pregnancy without some stomach upset. It may be true morning sickness with nausea or vomiting, or it may be an uneasy, burning, gassy feeling in your stomach. The first approach to eliminating or reducing indigestion, heartburn and gas is the same as the treatment of morning sickness. Eat smaller, more frequent meals; avoid foods that are irritating and cause distress such as fried or highly spiced foods; eat more bland foods and drink more milk.

If that doesn't do the trick, an occasional tablespoon of an antacid liquid or an antacid tablet is probably harmless. You may recall from the last chapter that one study did suggest an increased incidence of birth defects in women who took large amounts throughout pregnancy, but it is unlikely (although not studied at all) that occasional use will harm the unborn child (see refs. Chapter 9). There is one caution. Antacids containing sodium, such as Alka-Seltzer, may give too much salt and lead to fluid retention. The ones to take are those that contain aluminum hydroxide, magnesium trisilicate or magnesium hydroxide, alone or in combination. Maalox, Gelusil, Amphogel, Milk of Magnesia are some representative brands.

Backache

Backache is a common symptom in pregnancy. Sometimes it occurs very early, and some patients may get a series of X rays to evaluate back pain before they realize that they are pregnant. Be cautious about having X rays if it is at all possible that you might be pregnant—a subject we'll cover at length in Chapter 18.

Back pain may simply be due to pressure and stretching of the growing baby, or it can mean something more serious. Ruptured discs or kidney infections can give those symptoms, and serious problems like those demand medical attention.

If you and your doctor decide that the backache is simply due to some stretching, or straining of muscles or ligaments, so common in pregnancy, try some simple measure. A board under your mattress, more rest, a heating pad, or a light maternity girdle may be all you need. If you must take some pain medication, a small amount of codeine may be safer than aspirin. If you and your doctor feel strongly that aspirin is called for, take as little as possible for as short a time as you can. Occasional judicious use, particularly long before delivery, is only slightly risky.

Abdominal Pains

Like backaches, abdominal pains may simply be a calling card of your growing baby, or they may be symptoms of a dangerous illness. Appendicitis, gall-bladder disease, intestinal blockage, ulcers—all may occur in the pregnant woman and all produce abdominal pain. So if you've got more pain in your belly than you think you should have, see your doctor. This is particularly important if you have vomiting, bowel changes or fever along with the pain in your abdomen.

Mild abdominal pain is most likely due to stretching of ligaments that attach to your uterus. It's only logical that the tremendous increase in your abdominal size is likely to produce some discomfort or even some pain. Rarely, if ever, will you need drugs for the abdominal discomfort that accompanies pregnancy. More rest, a soothing heating pad or a support girdle are the things to use.

Headache

Headaches, too, can come from harmless causes like tension, sinus problems, a cold, or, on the other hand, they can signify a serious problem. Mild, occasional headaches are of little concern (except that they make you uncomfortable), but persistent or severe headaches should be looked into. If your headaches are so bad that you are tempted to take some medication, call your doctor first. Try to do without aspirin or its substitutes. If you can't, occasional judicious use to help you over an acute episode of discomfort is probably relatively safe.

Hemorrhoids

If you had hemorrhoids before, they're likely to get worse when you're pregnant. If not, you may develop them. Hemorrhoids, an outpouching of veins that line the rectum, are prone to occur under the influence of the increased abdominal pressure that pregnancy brings.

Before using any drugs, see your doctor. Don't experiment with over-the-counter remedies. Warm soaks or mild stool softeners may be all you need. Your doctor may want to give you a gentle suppository containing glycerine and, perhaps, a local anesthetic. These are likely to be relatively safe, since the amount of drug is small. You'll want to use them for as short a period of time as possible, however. Drugs are absorbed quite well through the rectal lining. They can get into your blood and thus into the baby. There's currently no indication that local anesthetics used this way can harm the fetus, but there aren't any studies to prove that either. As always, the safest practice is no drugs if possible. So use these suppositories if you need them, but stop using them as soon as you practically can. It's hard for you to tell what is going on back there, so you'll have to let your doctor help you to decide.

Ideally, we would like to avoid operations during pregnancy, but hemorrhoids sometimes become intolerably large or bleed freely. If that happens your doctor may recommend an operation, and you may have no choice.

Fluid Retention

Swollen ankes, the most common sign of fluid retention, bothers most pregnant women. They frequently ask their doctors to help rid them of this annoying problem, usually because they don't like the way they look. All too often their doctors comply with their requests by prescribing diuretics or water pills.

In Chapter 9 we pointed out that the fluid and salt retention which occurs during pregnancy is normal and necessary. On rare occasion it can become massive and dangerous, or it can be associated with high blood pressure. Then drugs may be mandatory. Most often, for most pregnancies, the extra fluid that gathers is mother nature's way of being certain that the baby gets enough salts and water. If it is simply of cosmetic concern, or it only bothers you after you've spent the day on your feet, try another treatment: elevate your legs when you get the chance. Don't take drugs.

Fatigue

Fatigue and an excessive need to sleep are natural components of all pregnancies, most troublesome in the early months. Treat these with rest. Never succumb to the temptation to take pep-me-up pills like amphetamines or "uppers." Don't even fight your fatigue with a few extra cups of coffee. That's not a good idea either. We discuss why in Chapter 11.

Constipation

Sluggish, irregular or painful bowel movements often trouble pregnant women, particularly near the end of pregnancy. The best treatment, if it works, is to increase your intake of fruit juices, prunes and other natural laxatives. If it doesn't, you may have to take a mild laxative or stool softener. Ask your doctor for advice. Most of the gentle laxatives such as Colace, Milk of Magnesia, and Ex Lax are all right for short-term use. There is no indication that any of these harm the unborn child. Mineral oil should not be used. It can block absorption and rob you and your baby of certain essential fat-soluble vitamins.

Vaginal Discharge

Leukorrhea, the medical term for a vaginal discharge, is common in pregnancy. Usually it is a normal response of the body to hormonal changes of pregnancy. When it is, there is no specific treatment. Occasionally, if it becomes too annoying you might use a very mild douche, but do this only after your doctor has advised you to do so and instructed you how. Douching during pregnancy, if not done properly, can be dangerous.

At times leukorrhea may be due to an infection. Most common are the protozoa *Trichomonas,* the fungi *monilia,* and the bacteria *Gonococcus.* Gonorrhea, the infection caused by *Gonococcus,* invariably needs to be treated (see Chapter 12). The others are extremely common and generally don't need to be treated unless the symptoms become severe.

If burning, itching or pain in the vaginal area is intense due to *Trichomonas* or *Monilia,* your doctor may want to treat you with an antiseptic douche or suppository. To date we know of no harmful side effects on the unborn child from short-term use of these agents. So, if your only problem is a mild symptomatic discharge due to harmless organisms, no treatment is the best approach. If, on the other hand, you've got real problems—either a bad bug or severe symptoms —you'll need a course of drug therapy. Your doctor will be able to take a culture and prescribe appropriate therapy, if needed.

Summary

1. Pregnant women suffer from a variety of bothersome physical problems, including various aches and pains, fatigue, hemorrhoids, fluid retention, morning sickness, indigestion and many more.
2. Most of these are problems you can live with. They may be uncomfortable, but they are minor and self-limited.
3. Don't ever treat yourself with drugs. Try not to ask your doctor for drugs unless you are so uncomfort-

able that you just have to get relief. Keep in mind that when it comes to these minor complaints of pregnancy, your request is often the key factor that determines whether or not you are given some medication. Your doctor is the one who makes the final decision, but often he can only judge the need by what you tell him and, perhaps, by how demanding you are. He may reason, "chances are it won't hurt the baby, and I'll keep my patient happy."

4. Pregnant women can get serious illnesses which must be treated with drugs. In cases like these, your doctor will let you know what he thinks you need and why. We'll discuss some of these more serious problems in Chapter 12.

XI

Stimulants
and Depressants

Now we return to that smoking, martini-sipping new-born we met in Chapter 1. The image may be somewhat exaggerated, but there's more truth in it than you might imagine.

You've now begun to realize that the unborn child gets his share of all those things that you swallow or inhale out of habit or need—that wake-up cup of coffee, the after-meal cigarette, the five-o'clock scotch and soda unwinder and all the other uppers and downers that help you get through your day. All of them are drugs that somehow alter your internal functions. Many act on your brain and change its messages. By so doing they affect perception, mood and those nebulous parts of your inner self we call the "mind" and "spirit."

The baby's mind before birth is a secret, mysterious world, hidden from our view. We know that much of the basic brain machinery exists quite early in prenatal life: the nerve pathways, the collections of tightly packed control centers, and the chemical transmitters that move information from place to place. We also know that at age five months or so the fetus begins certain activities that require some nervous system control. He moves, opens his eyes, hears, perhaps sees, swallows, makes sucking motions, gasps for breath and may even suck his thumb.

Nicotine, caffeine, tranquilizers, amphetamines, and alcohol all affect adult nervous system functions. They all readily enter the tissues of the unborn child, and reason tells us that they must affect him as well.

Chronic exposure to certain mood-altering drugs can play havoc with the developing brain. Newborn babies of alcoholic or narcotic-addicted mothers are addicted themselves. But most mothers are not alcoholics or drug addicts. The major concern is with everyday drugs in everyday dosages. You probably would like to know whether a few doses of some potent pain medication, a couple of cups of coffee, the nicotine from half a pack of cigarettes or some occasional sleeping pills or tranquilizers might affect your growing baby. We worry about the adverse effects of these drugs on your unborn child, and as we progress in the chapter we will share with you whatever hard evidence currently exists about these dangers. But the answers, particularly about subtle behavioral or psychological effects are hard to pin down. They are far less concrete than a pathetic infant shaking violently in his first experience outside—cold-turkey narcotic withdrawal.

As we said in Chapter 8, it is even hard to show that a drug causes a gross deformity. Proving that drugs like caffeine, nicotine or alcohol might cause behavioral changes in children is a monumental task. First of all, behavioral problems are hard to assess. They vary greatly, take time to develop, and don't leave telltale visible clues like the defects of missing arms, cleft palate, holes in the heart or misshapen ears. Next, if infants' emotional or behavioral problems do come from maternal smoking, coffee-drinking or use of alcohol, how do we prove it? After all, most women enjoy one or more of these social habits during pregnancy.

For these reasons, most studies to date have focused their attention on clear-cut injuries to the unborn child. Miscarriages, small birth weight, birth defects and death shortly after birth are the easiest to document. Only recently have some scientists made the first attempts to get at this elusive but vital question: does prenatal exposure to mind-altering drugs affect behavioral, psychological or social development?

Preliminary findings suggest that there may indeed be a variety of behavioral changes in offspring of women who took tranquilizers during their pregnancy.[1] The data is new and uncertain, but shocking nonetheless. And we may just be seeing the tip of the iceberg, for thousands of women in this country take a variety of mood-changing drugs throughout pregnancy. Moreover, if exposure to tranquilizers before birth may permanently alter psychological growth, what about those stimulants that are such a firm part of our social customs. Nicotine and caffeine are potent drugs, in many respects far more powerful than those tranquilizers studied.

Here is another observation which, at this point, is more philosophical than practical: in the past few years we have experienced an escalation of childhood behavioral problems. We have called this "hyperactivity" or "minimal brain dysfunction." One physician believes that an abundance of "food additives" is responsible. He claims that special additive-free diets "cure" these children. Others, who have studied the relationship to food additives in a more formal way, disagree. At this point we really don't know what makes these restless children behave the way they do. Could it be related to the increased use of cigarettes, coffee, alcohol and tranquilizers by modern women? Might they be affecting the immature brains of unborn children? We don't have the answer, but the possibility of such a cause is both real and alarming.

The effects of depressants and stimulants on the mental function, growth and maturation of unborn children, although of major concern, are difficult to pin down.

However, miscarriages, prematurity, low birth weight, birth defects, addiction, stillbirth and physical and mental blunting are much more visible effects. Some parts of the daily routine of many mothers are clearly guilty.

Smoking

It is always easiest to discuss something we know a lot about. The effect of maternal smoking on the unborn child has been studied extensively.[2-5]

Smoking, particularly more than 10 cigarettes per day, is a significant and proven risk factor in pregnancy. Both human and animal studies have shown a higher incidence of all of those hazards mentioned above in children of smoking mothers.

Many researchers have shown that smoking increases miscarriage rates, results in smaller babies and increases the incidence of prematurity.[2-8] Furthermore, the risk seems to increase in proportion to the number of cigarettes smoked.[9]

Some studies have found even more alarming effects of smoking. A group of British scientists looked at the long-term influences of prenatal exposure to smoking mothers. They found that children at age seven and later at eleven were shorter and intellectually slower in mathematics and reading when compared with offspring of nonsmoking women.[2] Subsequently, others have made similar observations.[10] It appears that mothers who smoke may be stunting both the physical and mental growth of their children.

The other frightening risk of maternal smoking is the likely increase in birth defects. Major birth defects, congenital heart diseases and cleft lip and palate seem to be more prevalent in children born of smoking mothers.[8,11-13]

No one knows what chemical component or consequence of cigarette smoking is responsible for these injuries. It may be the nicotine, carbon monoxide or cyanide, all of which are found in cigarette smoke; it may be a combination of those or some still unidentified factors. We haven't pinned down the cause, but we know that it's something in the smoke of cigarettes.

These aren't isolated or unconfirmed observations. They are well accepted and well researched. The inescapable conclusion: smoking during pregnancy is dangerous. Our advice is not to smoke while you are pregnant. If you can take that big step—STOP. If you can't stop, cut down. Remember, the dangerous effects are related to the number of cigarettes you smoke per day. Maybe this is the excuse you've been waiting for to quit.

Alcohol

Heavy alcohol consumption—let's say five beers or, a half-pint of whiskey per day—is disastrous to the unborn child. It causes a variety of birth defects, including heart, facial, arm and leg malformations.[14-17] Furthermore, infants of women addicted to alcohol are also addicted. They go through the same life-threatening withdrawal (D.T.s) after birth that alcoholics experience when they stop drinking.

Probably of far greater concern to you is the question of social drinking—a drink before dinner or an occasional two or three at a party. We really don't know where the dividing line is between social drinking and heavy drinking in terms of fetal malformations. We know that chronic alcoholic mothers pose a grave threat to their children, but no one has studied social drinkers in detail to see whether one drink a week, one per night, or two per night makes any difference.

It also is unknown, what, if any, psychological or mental impairment might result from exposing the fetus to alcohol. That infant in the carrier with a martini in hand is no different, not in the least, from your unborn child who has just shared your drink. Maybe it's all right to give your newborn baby a martini—we really don't know that either—but most of you would be shocked at that suggestion. If you keep that picture in mind when you're at a party, you might, at least, keep the alcohol intake down.

The final analysis of social drinking is that it's probably okay to have a drink or two a week, but if you can readily do without alcohol for those nine months, it's a good idea to abstain, since we just don't know how the fetus is influenced.

Coffee

A few studies have found a higher incidence of birth defects in animals exposed to caffeine before birth.[18-20] The dosages were always high—much greater than you would get from your daily three cups of coffee. Human studies have not raised a flag of caution, at least as far as birth defects are concerned. But birth defects are not our sole worry.

Coffee and tea are potent stimulants. Tea contains as much caffeine as coffee does. Caffeine has powerful effects on the central nervous system and on many other sites of the body. It places almost every organ in a state of readiness, wound up for full activity. It does this, at least in part, by blocking the action of a certain enzyme whose function is to break down a chemical messenger. When that enzyme is inhibited or stopped by caffeine, the messenger stays around in high concentration.

This particular messenger, known as cyclic AMP, is found everywhere in the body. It carries out a vast number of functions, such as helping hormones such as insulin, thyroid hormone and cortisone to work, helping cells to secrete and absorb various substances, and assisting the fledgling cells of the blastocyst and embryo to differentiate into proper organs. Cyclic AMP, it seems, may be one of the most vital substances common to all animal life.

Why do we go into these technical details? Because we are concerned about the possible consequences of persistent high levels of caffeine on the unborn child. To a scientist, it seems inconceivable that chronic stimulation of a chemical as important as cyclic AMP wouldn't have some adverse, or at least unnatural influence on this tiny growing being. Caffeine readily enters its tissues. And if you are like most Americans, you drink a lot of coffee. Therefore, you continually bombard your baby's vulnerable organ systems with a potent chemical that has known, drastic physiological and chemical effects on the human body. The effects of coffee are more pronounced than those of moderate smoking or alcohol consumption.

Switch to decaffeinated coffee if you possibly can. If you can't switch, keep your regular coffee or tea consumption to an absolute minimum. The potency and widespread effect of caffeine markedly alter the fetal environment. Should you, or *need* you, tamper with nature that drastically?

Tranquilizers

Tranquilizers, as the name implies, are drugs that help calm jangled nerves. They alter mood by reducing tension. There are many types of tranquilizers. Some are quite potent and are generally reserved for people with serious psychiatric problems. Those are the so-called "major tranquilizers" or phenothiazines. Thorazine, Sparine, Mellaril are some examples. For most of you the minor tranquilizers are of much greater interest, since your doctor is likely to prescribe them for mild tension and everyday nervousness or anxiety.

The most commonly used "minor tranquilizers" fall into two chemical classes: benzodiazepines and meprobamate. If these sound like mouthfuls, their common names will probably be more familiar. Valium and Librium are the main benzodiazepines. Miltown and Equanil are the most common brands of meprobamate.

Chances are good that you or someone you know has taken one of these drugs at one time or another. The Health Research Group found that 31.7 million prescriptions for Valium alone were written in 1975; 5.6 million were for women of the childbearing ages 20–39. Prescriptions for Miltown, Equanil and related tranquilizers totaled 3.6 million including 400,000 in the 20–39 group of women.[21]

In view of these staggering numbers there is little wonder that health care specialists, particularly those concerned with the well-being of the unborn child, have finally begun to ask: "What effect do these drugs have on the fetus?"

Once again, the main focus of investigation has been fetal deformities. Behavioral problems have not been scrutinized to any great extent. The results of the studies are conflicting. Some have shown that both of these classes of minor tranquilizers do predispose to birth defects, if the drugs are taken during the first trimester of pregnancy.[22-24] Some studies have come to opposite conclusions—they have not identified an associated rise in malformations.[25]

At this point the positive studies exceed the negative ones in quality and number. Moreover, as we have warned many times before, any positive findings are cause for caution, particularly when the need or benefit of a drug is low. The FDA agrees and has recently issued the following warning:

While these data do not provide conclusive evidence that minor tranquilizers cause fetal abnormalities, they do suggest such an association.

Since use of these drugs during the first trimester of pregnancy is rarely a matter of urgency, benefit-risk considerations are such that their use during this period should almost always be avoided.[26]

There's that risk/benefit concept that we've spoken of many times before. In this case, the risk (at least of fetal deformities) is suggested, but not absolutely proven. Moreover, it probably isn't enormous. Surely, if you take these drugs you don't run a 50 percent or even a 10 percent chance of having a deformed child. But the risk, however small, may be two to eight times greater than if you didn't take the drugs.

How about the benefit? These are relatively mild drugs, usually used for slight degrees of nervousness, tension and anxiety. In most cases they aren't essential. Can it be that six million women in that 20–39 age group can't do without these mild calmatives? We very much doubt it. For most women there's just not enough benefit to justify the risk. Another note of caution: the studies that have identified these apparent hazards to fetal development point to the first trimester, the time of maximum organ formation, as the riskiest time. Remember, for the first part of that first trimester most of you won't know you are pregnant. So if there's any chance that you might become pregnant, try to avoid these drugs.

Other studies have looked at the possible hazards of tranquilizers when they are given to the mother near delivery time and when they are used chronically throughout pregnancy in large dosages. Some have suggested that exposed newborns are depressed. Their breathing, other body functions and muscle tone aren't as strong as those of unexposed babies. Finally, a few youngsters seemed to be addicted and developed delayed signs of drug withdrawal when their mothers took minor tranquilizers throughout pregnancy.[27-29] As before, subtle, long-term changes in behavior and mental function in exposed children are hard to assess and have only recently been investigated. Those studies mentioned earlier in this chapter do suggest that prenatal exposure to tranquilizers may be a negative influence on childhood behavior and psychological development.[1]

Narcotics

Narcotics are potent pain killers. They are also euphoriants, mood elevators and depressants that are widely abused in today's drug culture. Morphine, Demerol, codeine, Dilaudid, heroin, opium, Percodan, propoxyphene (Darvon) and pentazocine (Talwin) are some familiar legal and illegal members of the narcotic family.

If you have a problem while you are pregnant that produces severe pain, your doctor may want to give you one of these drugs. Such conditions are generally short-lived. An unbearable toothache, a migraine headache, a sprain or fracture, pain after an operation, are some examples that come to mind.

There is no evidence to date that short-duration use of appropriate dosages of narcotics is harmful to the unborn child. Just be sure to tell the treating physician that you are pregnant (or might be). In this instance, therefore, the benefit may exceed the known or suspected risks. If your pain is unbearable, by all means get the relief you need. Just try to get off of these potent drugs as soon as possible.

There are two other times when narcotics that are not as safe for the unborn child are used by mothers. They include the chronic, excessive abuse by addicts, and the very common administration in labor and delivery.

The horrors of narcotic addiction are vividly etched in your minds by movies and TV shows. You have seen them "shooting up" and going "cold turkey." You have seen them overdosed and rushed to emergency rooms. It's obvious that this must spell disaster for the unborn child—miscarriages, prematurity and stillbirths are common ends of pregnancies of addicted mothers.[30,31] The infants that do survive are generally born addicted, and saving their lives is a major medical challenge.[30,32]

The final serious concern about narcotics in pregnancy comes from their extensive use in labor and delivery. These are depressant drugs, so babies exposed shortly before birth are less active, don't breathe as well and are often cyanotic (blue) for longer periods than unexposed newborns (see ref. Chapter 13). The implications of this are important and will be considered in more detail in Chapter 13.

Barbiturates

"Yellow jackets," "rainbow pills," "red devils," and scores of other nicknames have followed these drugs into the streets. When used properly, they are marvelous aids to modern medical treatment. They calm distraught individuals; bring needed rest to those who would otherwise toss and turn; lull you to sleep before a major operation; reduce out-of-control blood pressure, and they help patients with epilepsy to overcome the crippling of grand mal seizures.

When they are used in excess or without medical guidance, these "wonder drugs" become vicious killers that trap and destroy their victims. The barbiturate addict is unable to function effectively, for the drug brings chronic depression, lack of energy and loss of concentration. Worse, the addict can't stop taking the drug, for the withdrawal symptoms are far worse than those from heroin. Death from barbiturate withdrawal is common. This scene is obviously no place for a growing embryo or fetus. The offspring of barbiturate addicts often don't survive the pregnancy. If they do, the drug withdrawal that awaits them—for they are born addicted—is frequently too much for their tiny bodies to endure.

Some of you may need to take barbiturates while you are pregnant for valid medical reasons. You may need them only for a brief while—for example before an operation, or to help you sleep during a short hospital stay. Or you may need them throughout, for example to control epileptic seizures. We talk about these indications and what this may mean to you and your unborn child in Chapter 12. Short-term use is probably quite safe. Long-term use, in epileptics, may be associated with a somewhat increased incidence of birth defects, but the risk is quite low. So, if there is strong medical indication, by all means take these drugs with medical guidance and supervision. The benefit to you and your unborn child outweighs the small risk.

Amphetamines

These potent central nervous system stimulants should never be taken during pregnancy. Unlike barbiturates, which have important medical uses, amphetamines are used for only two reasons, weight control, and, as abused drugs for the exhilaration they bring. Pregnant women should not be taking drugs to control weight. And the illicit use of amphetamines to get "high" is far too dangerous for anyone, particularly for someone who is responsible for an unborn child.

Amphetamines readily cross the placenta and enter the baby's body. They are potent stimulants that have profound effects on the brain. We don't know what their long-term effects are, but it would be most surprising if they didn't leave indelible psychological scars on the unborn child.

We do know that amphetamines can produce birth defects. Animal studies have convincingly shown this.[33,34] Studies in humans, while less certain, have also related a variety of birth defects to their chronic use by mothers.[35-37] Amphetamines, then, are on the list of never-to-be-taken drugs. This applies to everyone at all times, but is doubly true for the pregnant woman.

Marijuana

We don't know very much about the effects of marijuana on the unborn child. Too bad, since this may well be a drug that you want to know something about. A number of animal studies have identified a variety of birth defects when animals were exposed to marijuana extract, to the smoke or to the active agent, THC.[38-40] Human studies are still too few to draw any firm conclusions. We don't yet know whether the frequency of birth defects is increased when mothers smoke marijuana. We do know that many women who have smoked this drug have given birth to seemingly normal children.

The other thing we don't know is what effect, if any, this drug has on the developing brain. If you smoke marijuana, you know what it does to you and your perceptions. Only you can decide whether you want to expose your unborn child to such alteration in brain function. The same recommendation that we gave about alcohol applies here: stop if you can. If not, at least keep your use of this drug to a bare minimum.

LSD, Mescaline and Other Hallucinogens

Many animal studies have associated birth defects with maternal exposure to these drugs.[41,42] Human data is less certain, although some surveys have found a higher incidence of congenital defects in children of LSD users.[43,44] The effects of these drugs on physiological and psychological function is quite profound—much more marked than small amounts of alcohol or marijuana. The effect on the unborn child? Again, no one knows.

Our strong inclination would be to recommend that you stay away from these while you are pregnant. There are two reasons. First of all, drugs which are so strong and potentially dangerous for you are likely to be bad for your tiny unborn child. Secondly, these drugs are sold illegally, and they are often adulterated with quinine or other materials. You really don't know what you are getting. Even if the LSD were safe for your unborn child, the stuff it's mixed with might be deadly.

Summary

In this chapter we have discussed those common drugs, legal and illegal, that may be part of your daily routine. They may help pry open your sleepy eyes, give you a feeling of well-being or relax your jangled nerves. Amphetamines, barbiturates, LSD and marijuana may be strangers to you, but cigarettes, coffee and alcohol are more likely to be parts of your daily routine. You may light up or sip them without giving a second thought. We want to remind you that if you are pregnant, you are a new mother. You carry inside you for a brief but critical time a forming baby. What you take into your body can no longer be done thoughtlessly.

The lesson this chapter brings: if you can, do without or with less alcohol, nicotine, caffeine, tranquilizers and other mind-altering drugs. Ask yourself: would I give this coffee, this cigarette, this alcoholic drink or this pill to my baby? Let the answer guide the handling of that even-more-vulnerable not yet born fetus.

XII

Drugs for
Serious Illnesses

Drugs aren't always bad for you and your unborn child. They may be lifesaving in times of painful or treacherous illness. In the group of "treacherous illnesses" we will include illnesses that can threaten your health, as well as those that present little danger to you but are a major threat to your unborn baby.

For numerous acute and chronic conditions drugs are "just what the doctor ordered." We advised you when not to take medicines; we should also tell you some of the times when you can and must.

Acute illnesses strike suddenly and leave just as briefly as they came. A few visits to the doctor, a brief hospital stay, an uncomplicated operation, and a week or two of medications usually allay them. The most common acute illnesses are infections. These are intrusions into our body by invisible invaders that we commonly call "bugs," which come in many sizes, shapes and biological forms. They include viruses, bacteria, parasites such as worms and protozoa, and fungi.

Infections can strike any organ in the body. They can affect you and make you so ill you'll be forced to call your doctor, or, they may be deceivingly mild: a slight bit of nausea, a very short-lived rash, a minor vaginal discharge or sore—something you barely notice, yet something that can be devastating for your unborn child.

126

A pregnant woman has no special armor. You are just as vulnerable to infection as anyone else. And if you get one you might have to take an antibiotic drug to wipe it out.

Injuries are acute illnesses. You may be in an automobile accident and find yourself the recipient of a broken bone or two or the unlucky victim of an internal injury that requires an operation. You may need general anesthesia (drugs) while the bones are set or the internal injuries are patched up. You may need pain medications (more drugs) after the operation or even for the agonizing pain that may accompany severe bruises.

Should you develop an acute dental problem while you are pregnant, the dentist may need to take X rays (generally a no-no while you are pregnant); may want to give you a local anesthetic (a drug) to deaden the pain while he drills or pulls, or may want to put you to sleep with an intravenous sedative or a gas that you inhale (drugs again).

Suppose you awaken one morning with a sharp pain in the lower right side of your abdomen—you guessed it: appendicitis. General anesthesia and an operation followed by a week of pain medications may be essential. Pregnant women do, at times, need operations, not only for appendicitis, but for gallbladder disease, ruptured ulcers, intestinal blockage and others. Drugs and more drugs may be vital in your fight toward a successful recovery.

Pregnant women may also have chronic illnesses. These are conditions that last for months or years preceding or developing during your pregnancy. They may need constant treatment or lie dormant, smoldering under the surface, waiting to erupt without warning. They may be mild like a minor rash or potentially fatal like leukemia. The list of chronic illnesses fills 10-pound text books of internal medicine, so we'll just mention some of the more common ones, particularly those that you, a young woman, might face. High blood pressure, asthma, seizures (epilepsy), blood clots in the legs (phlebitis), and diabetes are among the most prevalent.

Acute Illnesses

Infections

Bacteria, minute one-celled organisms, are responsible for many of our infections. To fight them we use a variety of antibiotics and antibacterial drugs. Even though you are pregnant you may sometimes have to take these drugs, since the infection, if left untreated, may spread out of control. The golden rule, as we've discussed many times, is to weigh the risk against the benefit. The single, safest bacteria fighter likely to be effective is the one to take. Infections aren't all the same. Some are far more serious than others. You wouldn't chase a fly with a shotgun; nor should your doctor treat a minor bladder infection with a powerful and potentially dangerous antibiotic (kanamycin, for example) when equally effective, milder ones could do the trick. Conversely, you wouldn't try to ward off an attacking lion with a flyswatter, nor should your doctor hesitate to treat aggressively a serious infection. A potent, but potentially dangerous antibiotic may be mandatory if your life is threatened by meningitis, bacteria in the bloodstream, peritonitis or a massive pneumonia. In cases like these you accept whatever risk is necessary to effect the quickest cure.

As a rule, the treatment of infections is best guided by information from a bacterial culture. You've probably experienced this when your doctor took a culture of your or your child's throat to tell whether that redness and pain was caused by the *Streptococcus* bacteria (the familiar "strep throat"). Doctors can sample many sites of suspected infection—the throat to look for a strep infection; the urine to tell whether the bladder or kidney is infected; the sputum to check for a pneumonia, or the stool to evaluate an intestinal infection. The laboratory grows the bacteria and tests for antibiotic sensitivity. This gives your doctor two valuable pieces of information. First, is there or is there not an infection caused by bacteria? Second, if there is, how can it best be treated? His next step is to choose the safest drug that is likely to work.

Sometimes your doctor may want to give you an antibiotic without taking a culture or before the culture results come back from the laboratory (it generally takes two days). There are times when this is justified. You may have a red, nasty-looking throat and a high fever. The diagnosis: strep, until proven otherwise, and a course of penicillin may be in order. If you have an obvious pneumonia, seen on chest X ray or detected by physical examination, starting antibiotics before the sputum culture comes back from the laboratory may be in your best interest. Finally, you may have a very grave infection such as peritonitis, meningitis or bacteria in the bloodstream. It would be foolish to delay emergency treatment while the laboratory worked on your cultures.

Infections of the Urinary Tract— Cystitis (Bladder Infections) and Pyelonephritis (Kidney Infections)

As many as 10 out of every 100 pregnant women develop an infection of the urinary tract. These may go unnoticed if they don't cause any discomfort, and the only indication that an infection is present comes from the routine urine examinations in your doctor's office. Other times you may have classic symptoms of burning and pain on urination, increased frequency of urination, a sensation of fullness in the bladder or the more serious symptoms of back pain and fever.

The high rate of urinary infections in pregnant women is due, in part, to mechanical changes that go along with pregnancy. The growing uterus distorts the bladder, which lies directly in front of it. This distortion can cause urine to collect and never be completely eliminated. Stagnant urine, like a stagnant pool of water, is fertile territory for bacterial growth; the result: a bladder infection or cystitis. This infection, if untreated, can then spread up the ureters (the tubes that connect the bladder to the kidneys) and infect the kidneys.

Most authorities urge prompt treatment of all urinary

tract infections. The drugs most commonly used are ampicillin (a type of penicillin), sulfonamides and nitrofurantoins. All of these antibacterial drugs are relatively safe for the unborn child, the safest being ampicillin, which is also the most effective and the one most often used. How fortunate that you can take these with an easy mind, since the chances are one in 10 that you may have to do so.

Infections of the Lungs—Pneumonia

Pneumonias, infections of the lungs, are also quite common, but not nearly as frequent as urinary tract infections. When pregnant women get pneumonia there are special difficulties, again due to the growing uterus. During pregnancy you may, at one time or another, have bolted upright in bed, unable to catch your breath. Pressure on the diaphragm by the enlarging uterus is one of the reasons. Pneumonia can impair normal breathing even further; hence the pregnant woman, her breathing reserves already stretched, is more vulnerable to the dangers of a lung infection.

Urgent treatment, for the sake of both her and her unborn child, is imperative, since their oxygen supply can become critically low. Antibiotics are often needed, and your doctor may make an educated guess in choosing the one he feels is most appropriate. Later, he may make a change after sputum-culture results give more accurate guidance. Fortunately, as with urinary tract infections, the most common pneumonias can be treated with relatively safe antibiotics, and a rapid cure can be found without jeopardizing your unborn child.

Infections of the Genital Tract (VD)— Gonorrhea ("Clap"), Syphilis

Gonorrhea

Gonorrheal infection is a serious threat to the newborn. As the baby leaves his mother's body he can contract the disease. The most vulnerable targets are his eyes which can be engulfed by infection and blinded forever. Eyedrops of silver nitrate are now routinely given to babies in hospitals to help prevent this dreadful complication, but they aren't foolproof. Moreover, for babies born at home or on the way to the hospital, the drops may be overlooked. Consequently, gonorrhea during pregnancy must be found, treated and, if possible, eradicated before the baby can be exposed. The penicillins, the class of drugs usually used, are thought to be safe. Occasionally, the bacteria may be resistant to this drug and tetracyclines, another group of antibiotics, must be substituted. This drug is more hazardous to the fetus for reasons that will be discussed shortly.

One problem with gonorrhea is detection. Quite likely a woman doesn't know that she has it. The severe abdominal and pelvic pain that often occurs in nonpregnant women, due to infection of the tubes and ovaries, rarely happens in pregnancy. The only symptoms may be some vaginal burning or itching or a suspiciously heavy discharge. If you get any of these, a hasty trip to the doctor is in order.

Syphilis

To many of you, syphilis may seem a distant memory —a disease that ended sometime in the Middle Ages, perhaps, or with Columbus? Not so! Syphilis is alive and well and it's on the upsurge, just as gonorrhea is. More and more frequently, people who catch one, catch the other. Not only is it increasing at an alarming rate, but it also is a nightmare for the unborn child. It is one of the very few bacteria that can actually cross the placenta and enter the body of the growing fetus. When it does, it leaves a path of destruction: death before delivery or a life of misery. The many faces of congenital syphilis include infection of every organ, severe anemias, mental retardation, blindness, deafness and facial distortion.

The only sure way of avoiding this silent killer is by minimizing exposure. Syphilis is a venereal disease that is transmitted from person to person through sexual intercourse. The fewer the contacts, the less the likelihood of getting the disease. But accidents will happen and you may contract syphilis. If you do, early treatment with penicillin can cure both you and your baby. If caught early enough, the chances are very good that your baby won't suffer any ill effects from the disease. The big problem is that syphilis is even sneakier than gonorrhea: most often, you have no idea that you have been infected. Occasionally you may notice a small sore in your genital area, but more often there are no telltale signs. A deformed baby may be the first visible calling card of the disease.

Before you throw up your hands in despair, there is one salvation. A simple blood test can tell whether or not you have syphilis or have had it in the recent past. All women should have this test as soon as they become pregnant, and at regular intervals thereafter to avoid the lifelong heartache of a syphilitic child.

Urinary tract infections, pneumonia and the venereal diseases, gonorrhea and syphilis, are but a few of the many infections the pregnant woman may get. They all share a single golden rule of treatment, particularly when you are pregnant: the severity of the illness for you and your baby must determine the potency of the drugs used. You and your doctor can tell how sick you are, or how threatened your baby is, and whether a dangerous drug may be needed.

If your illness requires it, you may decide to seek the care of a doctor or a specialist other than your obstetrician. You must remember to tell any doctor whom you are seeing that you are pregnant. Keep in mind that although he or she is a doctor, that person may not necessarily be well-versed in the care of pregnant women. An unborn baby and its mother are special kinds of patients. Thus, it might be a good idea to have this doctor consult with your obstetrician about your diagnosis and treatment, if any becomes necessary.

To help you share intelligently in the discussions and decisions you and your doctor will make, let's just discuss a few of the more common drugs used to treat bacterial infections. You owe it to yourself and your unborn child to learn as much as you can about those drugs which might enter your body and that of the baby inside you, too. You are now responsible for two lives; the information that follows can vitally affect the future of both. Once you have some idea of the risks involved, you can, along with your doctor, decide whether to take that chance.

Antibacterial Drugs*

Antibacterial drugs help the body's own defenses to destroy those dangerous invaders. The familiar antibiotics are only one class of these antibacterial drugs. To be called an "antibiotic," the drug must actually be made by another living organism, generally a fungus or mold. Penicillin, tetracycline, erythromycin, streptomycin are some examples. Other drugs, like the nitrofurantoins and the sulfas, are useful in combatting certain bacterial infections, but they are not antibiotics. They are man-made chemicals.

Penicillins

Most penicillins, including the very common relative ampicillin, are familiar to all of you. They were among the first antibiotics discovered, and they are still the most useful and most widely used. As far as we know they are safe for the unborn child. Yet there remains an aura of uncertainty, for although these drugs are used by the truckloads for everyone including pregnant women, only a few inadequate studies have analyzed their effects on the unborn child. All we have is our impression and suspicion that they are relatively safe. This means that if you truly need to take penicillins while you are pregnant, you can do so with fair confidence that your child will be unaffected. But don't take them without your doctor's agreement, or for illnesses like the common cold, which they don't cure. They are still drugs—foreign chemicals for your unborn child. Remember that their subtle effects on these maturing tissues have never been fully explored.

Streptomycin and Related Drugs
(Neomycin, Kanamycin, Gentamicin)

These are all potent antibiotics with well-known hazards and side effects. The kidneys and the inner

*Drugs have many different names, depending upon the company which produces them. Therefore, you should ask your doctor not only the name of the drug, but the category to which it belongs. We will discuss and list the drugs below by category.

ear are the targets of their toxic attacks. Permanent dizziness, hearing loss and kidney failure can result from treatment with these drugs, particularly if large doses are taken over a long period. The unborn child takes up these drugs and is sensitive to their destructive effects. Exposed newborns have been born deaf or with kidneys that wouldn't work. Unlike penicillin, streptomycin and its relatives must be reserved for the gravest of situations. This is true for anybody, but doubly so for the pregnant woman.

Most of these drugs need to be given by injection; they don't come in pill form. Most are used only in the hospital. This means that there is little chance that you will come across any of these unless you are sick enough to be in a hospital.

If your doctor wants to give you one of these, make sure you know why. Let's take an example: you have a severe kidney infection; your doctor takes a urine culture and the laboratory reports that the bacteria are sensitive to both ampicillin and gentamicin. You should probably be given ampicillin (unless you are allergic to penicillin) rather than the other, more dangerous drug.

At times, the threat of the infection may far outweigh the risk of taking the drug. If so, take it. If it is used cautiously, in the lowest possible dosage and for the shortest possible time, there is small chance that your unborn child will be harmed. The choice of a drug and the dangers it presents are things that you and your doctor should discuss. Remember, when you ask questions of your doctor, you do so for the sake of your baby, not for the purpose of challenging your doctor's authority or medical expertise. If the choice of antibiotic has been well-founded, your doctor will welcome your questions as a concerned mother.

Tetracyclines

Next to the penicillins, these antibiotics are used most often. Because they are quite safe for adults they are frequently used with reckless abandon, very often for conditions that don't call for antibiotics. For the unborn child they are a known hazard.

They have the unique tendency to adhere tightly to the calcium of growing bones, and the baby's bone growth will be significantly slowed while you are taking the drug. If the drug is given for an appropriate illness over a brief period, the slowing of your baby's bone growth will only be temporary. However, if you take tetracycline daily or often to keep your skin clear, stop it during your pregnancy.

Growth of bones, and particularly teeth, is most active during the last half of intrauterine life. An unborn child exposed to tetracycline during this period of tooth formation may carry with him a lifelong scar. Staining of permanent teeth, ranging from a slight tinge to an obvious unsightly brown, is a common aftermath. If possible, avoid these drugs during the last half of pregnancy. There usually are equally effective and far less harmful substitutes.[2]

Chloramphenicol

Chloramphenicol is another antibiotic that presents a known risk to the unborn child. A newborn whose mother is given this drug just before delivery may show symptoms of, or even die from the "gray-baby syndrome." Chloramphenicol passes easily into the baby where it soon rises to dangerously high concentrations for, unlike his mother, his immature protective devices cannot get rid of the drug. In these high concentrations the drug interferes with the newborn's breathing. He literally suffocates, becomes blue or gray; hence, the name "gray-baby syndrome."[3]

The drug also poses other serious hazards for the mother. Therefore, most physicians today use it only for very special and serious infections. Typhoid fever is one. Avoid this drug unless your physician can assure you that it is your only hope. Especially keep away from it near your due date. You don't want a gray baby.

Other Antibiotics

Many other antibiotics, including clindamycin, cephalosporins, lincomycin, erythromycin have not been well tested for possible hazard to the unborn child. If a better-known antibiotic like penicillin will do just as well, it's wiser to stick with that one. We know more about it. If there isn't any choice, you may have to take one of these others. To date, there is no cause for alarm if you do. Although large-scale studies don't exist, individual experiences have been encouraging. Many pregnant women have taken all of these with no apparent ill effects on the child.

Sulfa Drugs (Sulfonamides)

Chances are fairly high that you may be given one of these during your pregnancy. They are commonly used for urinary tract infections, a frequent foe of pregnant women. They do not seem to present a danger to the unborn child. If they do cause any difficulties—birth defects in particular—it can't be very often. Literally thousands of pregnant women who have taken sulfonamides are proud mothers of happy, healthy children.

There is one concern. In Chapter 7 we discussed the many adverse effects that drugs can have on the unborn or newborn infant. One was an alteration in normal bilirubin metabolism with resulting jaundice (yellow skin coloration is the visible sign) and a serious condition known as "kernicterus." Kernicterus can lead to a permanent brain injury. It is probably due, in part, to accumulation of bilirubin in the brain itself. Sulfonamides, if present in the newborn, can produce this serious complication.[4,5] They do this rarely, and even exposed newborns generally fare quite well. But most physicians prefer to discontinue the sulfonamide treatment in advance of your delivery date. They reason: why take the chance of possibly damaging the vulnerable newborn?

If you have an infection that should be treated with sulfa drugs, go ahead and take them. You can be relatively confident that they won't hurt your unborn child. If you can stop them at least several days before delivery, however, so that your newborn is drug-free, it's a good idea to do so.

Nitrofurantoins

This is another group of antibacterial drugs that are commonly used to combat urinary tract infections, so you might run across them. Like sulfonamides, they are generally considered safe. The only known hazard is the very rare occurrence of severe neonatal anemia in certain susceptible newborns. Susceptibility is pretty well confined to black children who have a rather common congenital deficiency of a particular enzyme, glucose-6-phosphate dehydrogenase (G6PD). The current recommendation, then, is for black mothers to stop taking these drugs shortly before delivery. At other times, and for other individuals, there seems to be little risk to the unborn child.

Injuries

If you are severely injured, for example in an automobile accident, you may need an operation, the setting of a fracture, or at the very least some relief from the agonizing pain that may accompany severe bruises. We've asked you to try to endure minor aches and pains for the sake of your unborn child; minor problems aren't worth even slight risks. No one, on the other hand, would be so callous as to insist that you bear the pain of an operation, a bone manipulation, or even the miserable discomfort of bad bruises.

What can you do in these situations? And how safely? Strong pain medications, like narcotics, are probably relatively safe when taken in moderation for brief periods. We discussed the ravages of chronic drug addiction in Chapter 11, but that doesn't apply here. If you need some Demerol, morphine, codeine, Percodan or other potent pain killer, you can take them for a week or two. The overwhelming likelihood is that your unborn child will be unaffected. In fact, he may be more seriously harmed by the negative effects that excruciating pain may have on your body. Clearly, strong pain medications are sometimes essential; the only suggestion: stop them as soon as possible.

Aspirin and other mild pain killers are another matter. In general, if your aches and pains are slight enough to be controlled by these, you can probably do without them. The dangers these drugs can present have already been discussed in Chapter 9.

Dental Problems

Since this is a chapter about serious problems, let's first mention those dental situations that fit into this category. There are times when dental work is a must: a severe toothache, an abscess, infected gums, an impacted wisdom tooth producing pain and infection.

In general, most dental treatment is safe for your unborn child. As always, if he wants to give you an antibiotic, make sure it is the safest one possible. Your dentist will be less familiar with the possible hazards of antibiotics than your obstetrician will be. He might need an extra reminder that you are pregnant, a phone consultation with your doctor or perhaps some points that you've picked up from reading this chapter.

If you need an anesthetic, a local one is far safer than a general. If you must have additional sedation, a little nitrous oxide gas is far preferable to an intravenous barbiturate like pentothal. Intravenous drugs are more dangerous in general than nitrous oxide. They are more likely to depress your breathing and lower your blood pressure. If this happens, your unborn child can be in jeopardy.

If, for some reason, you must be deeply anesthetized, or if you have a major procedure, such as the extraction of impacted wisdom teeth, you should have this done in the hospital where a trained anesthesiologist can put you to sleep and keep a close eye on you.

What about those routine dental visits: the cleaning, regular checkups and filling cavities? These visits are needed and won't affect your unborn child.

The one routine dental procedure that we would question slightly while you are pregnant is full-mouth X rays. We realize that the radiation dosage in dental X rays is extremely low and the beam is localized to the mouth, far removed from your unborn child. Thus, the risk to him must be exceedingly small, but we don't know for certain whether even this minute amount of exposure might, on occasion, be harmful. If the machine is set wrong or malfunctions, you may then get more than you bargained for. Since you can generally get along for nine months without "routine" X rays of your mouth, it's probably a good idea to do so. If you have a toothache or any acute problem that requires X rays for proper diagnosis, however, by all means, let your dentist do what he must. The chances that this will be hazardous to your child are extremely remote.

Surgical Illnesses

Elective operations (ones that are not emergencies) such as repair of that "trick knee;" fixing your crooked nose; taking out a gallbladder that isn't working but isn't currently causing any trouble; removing a large, benign growth from your back should be postponed until after delivery. Urgent, life-threatening conditions cannot be put off.

Major surgical emergencies during pregnancy cause trouble for two reasons: they are often difficult to diagnose, and both the emergency itself and the operation can be serious blows to the unborn child.

Acute abdominal conditions such as cholecystitis, a gallbladder infection, which is somewhat more frequent in pregnant than in non-pregnant women, appendicitis, infected ovaries, bowel obstruction and all other abdominal conditions that potentially require surgery are far more difficult to diagnose in the pregnant woman. The pain that they may bring may not seem much different from the aches and pains of normal pregnancy. The elevation in the white blood cell count, so characteristic of an infection under usual circumstances, is frequently found in normal pregnancies. The tenderness, swelling and tightness of the abdominal wall—red flags to surgeons that trouble may be brewing—are identical to the usual pregnant abdomen. Finally, X rays, important diagnostic tools, can't be used as freely in pregnant women.

For all of these reasons, surgical emergencies involving abdominal conditions (far and away the most common kind) are hard to detect in the pregnant woman. This means that surgery may be delayed, and the chances that a problem may become more advanced before it is finally identified and treated are far greater in the pregnant woman. What can you do about this? Don't assume that every pain is a natural part of the pregnancy. If you get severe or new discomfort in your abdomen; if you get a fever or chills, contact your physician at once.

If it turns out that you have an acute surgical emergency, you may have to have an operation. If so, it is easier and safer to do it early in the course of the problem, since both you and your baby's lives are jeopardized by waiting for an appendix or gallbladder to rupture or for a twisted bowel to become gangrenous. The more severe the complications, the greater the risk to the unborn child. Thus, if you develop a serious problem like peritonitis, the chances of having a miscarriage are extremely high.

However, even uncomplicated operations during pregnancy carry a significant risk of miscarriage and premature labor. A gallbladder operation results in fetal death in approximately 25 percent of cases. An appendectomy, in approximately 15 percent.[6] Whether these unfavorable outcomes are due to the disease itself, the operative procedure, or the general anesthetic, is not known—it may be a combination of all three.

We do know that if you and your baby get through an abdominal operation successfully, you are probably home free. Studies performed to date indicate that babies who have survived maternal surgery do not have a higher incidence of birth defects.[6] The transient exposure to general anesthesia (unless there are complications like shock or poor oxygenation) does not predispose to birth defects. To sum up, serious surgery can be hazardous to the unborn child, but there's not much you can do about that except to get to the doctor at the first suggestion that something might be wrong. The earlier you get taken care of the better for both of you.

Chronic Illnesses

Hypertension (High Blood Pressure)

Pregnancy itself can produce hypertension, a condition known as "preeclampsia." Or you may be like thousands of others whose blood pressure is high for genetic reasons, because of some kidney or heart problems, or simply for reasons unknown. If your blood pressure is high, 140/90 or greater, you may need to take some medications. Untreated hypertension is no good for you or your baby, and the higher your blood pressure the worse the consequences.

The first drugs that your doctor is likely to give you for the high blood pressure are thiazide diuretics, commonly called "water pills." These not only rid your body of sodium and water, but they also relax the blood vessels and help to lower blood pressure. They are relatively mild drugs but often can take care of minor hypertension.

We've talked a bit before about them in Chapters 9 and 10. They are dispensed to pregnant women more frequently than almost any other drug, not to treat high blood pressure, but to get rid of some of the fluid that makes ankles swell. Unless this swelling is massive or potentially serious, diuretics should not be used, because this may produce undesirable salt and water imbalances for the growing fetus.

Another rare toxic effect of these drugs has been described. A few babies whose mothers were treated with these diuretic drugs were born with severe, occasionally fatal, deficiencies of their blood platelets (tiny cell-like globules in your blood that are needed for proper blood clotting).[7] When their number falls too low, bleeding results. Fortunately, this assault on the unborn child is extremely unusual. Moreover, these diuretics do not seem to cause developmental malformations in human beings.

Thus, if you have high blood pressure, you can take these drugs with fair assurance that they won't harm your unborn child. On the other hand, they shouldn't be used for a normal manifestation of pregnancy such as mild ankle swelling.

Other drugs are used for more severe hypertension, including methyldopa, reserpine, guanethidine, hydralazine and many others. If your blood pressure is so high that such potent drugs are required, you're better off being treated. They seem to be relatively safe. Many women have taken them with no ill effects on the unborn child. The only minor hazard that is known occurs with reserpine. Many babies who have been exposed to this drug near delivery choke and gasp from a strange sort of nasal congestion.[8] Most come through this okay, but a few have developed respiratory depression and died. It's advisable, therefore, to stop taking reserpine near your due date. If you still need a blood-pressure medication, see if your doctor can substitute one.

Asthma

If you suffer from asthma, your misfortune is the constant fear of being unable to breathe. When you have an attack your air passages clamp down, trapping the air inside your lungs and making every breath a painful, anxious experience. Severe asthma must be treated. You may have to take bronchodilating medications constantly throughout pregnancy, or if your attacks are intermittent, you may be able to get along with only occasional pills or whiffs from an inhaler. Although some experiments in animals have produced birth defects with these adrenaline-like drugs, human experience has not upheld this fear. Many asthmatic patients have taken drugs throughout pregnancy and have given birth to healthy, normal children.

As always, however, the best policy is no drugs if possible. If your asthma has not bothered you for many months and you take drugs "just to be safe," consult your doctor. You may be able to stop them while you are pregnant. If need be they can always be started again. Be on the watch, too, for circumstances that you know trigger an asthmatic attack: your neighbor's dog, or cat, or smoking. If at all possible, avoid them! It's worth the effort.

If your asthma is terribly severe, your doctor may be treating you with the most potent asthma fighters—corticosteroid drugs. Some reports have suggested higher incidences of fetal complications from these, including birth defects and prematurity.[9,10] If this is so, the incidence is rather low. A recent study of 70 women who took corticosteroids throughout pregnancy failed to note any serious risk to the unborn child. The recommendations from the study's authors was that if these drugs are strongly indicated they . . . "do not appear to noticeably increase the risk of maternal or fetal complications, and thus should not be contraindicated in pregnancy."[11] If you need potent medications to treat your asthma, you can take them with little fear that they will harm your unborn child.

Seizures (*Epilepsy*)

Epilepsy is one of the oldest afflictions of recorded medical history. The ancients ascribed the characteristic shaking, loss of consciousness or "fits" to possession by evil demons. We now have less supernatural explanations: epileptic seizures are caused by abnormal bursts of electrical activity that come from certain brain sites of the affected individual.

Seizure disorders range in intensity from mild lapses in memory, or the slight shaking of an extremity, to the full-blown loss of consciousness and convulsive shaking of the entire body that most people associate with this illness. You might think the problem is rare, since you probably have never seen anyone actually have an epileptic seizure. The truth of the matter is that seizure disorders are alarmingly common, but modern drug therapy is extremely effective. With proper treatment, those who suffer from this potentially debilitating or even life-threatening illness can lead near-normal lives.

Literally thousands of pregnant women in this country each year take antiseizure drugs; the most commonly used are Dilantin and phenobarbital. Those of you who do take drugs for seizure control may recently have read alarming reports about potential hazards to the unborn child. You have a right to know where you and your baby stand.

The evidence is now rather strong that birth defects are more common in children exposed to these drugs. It's somewhat difficult to identify relative risks of each of the drugs separately, since most patients take more than one at a time. Children born of mothers who take these drugs have approximately a three- to four-fold greater chance of having a birth defect than children born to mothers who did not take them.[12-15]

But before you throw up your hands in despair, if you are one of those women who takes one or more of these medications, let's see what this actually means. The chances of delivering a healthy baby are still strongly on your side. The probability that things will come out all right is in the order of 95 percent. Your baby's chances of having a birth defect (often minor, like cleft palate) are 4 percent to 6 percent, while the chances of drug-free babies having a defect are 1 percent to 2 percent.

This means, if you are a woman who has had a seizure problem, that you have two responsibilities. First, don't think that you must take the drugs automatically simply because you always have. Make sure you have a thorough evaluation to determine if the drugs are essential. If you are planning to become pregnant, see your doctor first; if you are already pregnant, make an appointment immediately.

Second, if you do have to take drugs to control seizures, don't worry. The chances that you will have a normal baby are overwhelmingly in your favor. Thousands of women before you who have been treated with these drugs have delivered healthy normal babies.

Blood Clots (Phlebitis)

Blood clots in the leg and pelvic veins are relatively common in pregnancy. In Chapter 7 we briefly mentioned the two drugs that can be used in this condition.

The easiest to use is the oral anticoagulant, commonly called a "blood thinner," coumarin. This drug crosses the placenta and gets into the baby's body and can cause probable birth defects when given in the first trimester, or fetal bleeding when the drug is given at other times, particularly close to delivery.[16, 17] If the activity of the drug is monitored very closely in the mother, it is relatively safe to the unborn child between months four and eight of the pregnancy. Even then, however, fetal bleeding can sometimes occur.

The alternative drug is heparin, which doesn't cross the placenta and has no known adverse effects on the fetus. Unfortunately, it is considerably harder to use, since it must be injected.

If you require anticoagulation while you are pregnant and can work out a way with your doctor to take heparin rather than coumarin, it's safer to do so. If your doctor wants to give you coumarin instead, be sure that your blood-clotting activity is closely monitored and try to avoid the drug in the earliest parts and the last month of pregnancy. Neonatal bleeding in infants exposed to the drug near delivery time is quite common and exceedingly dangerous.

Diabetes

Diabetes, particularly when severe, places a heavy burden on both the pregnant woman and the unborn child. The chances of fetal injury, including birth defects, death before birth or neonatal death are considerably greater in diabetic women.[18] Furthermore, pregnancy itself can make the diabetes worse.

Though the drugs themselves may confer some slight risk to the fetus, non-treatment seems to be far more dangerous. Women who are closely followed and treated properly and promptly have a far better chance of delivering a healthy child than women who neglect this serious problem.

Most authorities recommend using insulin rather than oral antidiabetic drugs during pregnancy. The outcome for mother and child are better when insulin is used, and the oral drugs are associated with a higher fetal complication rate.

If you are diabetic you need close, careful supervision throughout your pregnancy, preferably by an obstetrician who is well-versed in caring for women with your problem. You may have to take insulin even though you took no drugs or only oral drugs before. If you do, you can rest assured that this is the safest course for your unborn child. If your diabetes is sufficiently severe to require insulin, your child will fare far better if you take your shots than if you go through those nine months untreated.

Summary

You can see that even if you have some acute or chronic illness that may need drug treatment while you are pregnant, most of these problems can be handled with very little risk to you or your unborn child. Frequently, you must take medications for the good of both of you. To let a curable or treatable illness smolder, waiting to erupt may invite disaster. If you must take a drug or have an X ray, discuss the problem with your doctor. Make sure that he or she knows you are pregnant, or that you might be. Keep in mind that a vulnerable time for your unborn child is before you've even missed your first period. Therefore, even if you don't know you're pregnant but are trying to conceive or have been exposed, you may already be carrying a vulnerable being.

XIII

Drugs for Labor and Delivery

"Natural childbirth," the Lamaze method, the Bradley method, hypnosis, and now acupuncture capture the earnest attention of today's women. Why the interest in these methods? How do they differ from conventional practices? Which should you choose?

The thousands of women and their husbands breathing rhythmically and panting together in classes throughout the country concur with the apostles of these methods that "natural is better." Childbirth is not an illness, they say, but a normal and marvelous process, during which mothers should not be so groggy that they miss this wonderful event. Proponents of these natural methods have always believed that it made plain good sense not to fill the mother and her new baby full of drugs in those critical hours before birth. They've been laughed at and rejected by many members of the medical profession, but a minority has supported their "eccentricities" and helped those women who wanted to give birth "naturally."

Now you are faced with a decision: "Do I accept standard obstetrical techniques and any drugs that are offered? Is there any danger to me or my baby from the drugs used? Do I request some sort of modified drug regimen during labor and delivery? Or do I go 'natural' the whole way—no drugs at all?"

This is a deeply personal choice, and it's not one

which you can make quickly or take lightly. You may determine that natural childbirth is the only way for you; then, when the moment of reckoning actually arrives, you may find that your response to the pain simply won't let you go through with it. It certainly is not good for the new mother to feel she has failed and let herself, her husband and her new baby down because she needed some drugs during her delivery.

Natural childbirth is merely one method. It may be better, or at least safer, than modern obstetrical anesthesia techniques, but it isn't for everybody. To help you begin to make some choice, however, you need to know a few facts. How are babies normally delivered? Why is it better not to take drugs if you can avoid them? And, realistically, what are the risks if you opt for conventional drug-assisted labor and delivery?

You owe it to yourself and your unborn child to make that decision yourself. Don't let your doctor make it for you. Learn the pros and cons of each method, then decide.

American obstetrics has moved down a thoughtless and often dangerous path that Doris B. Haire, President of the International Childbirth Education Association has called "the Cultural Warping of Childbirth."[1] When anesthetic drugs were first used in the late 1800s to relieve some of the pain that accompanies the birth process, a new era in medicine was hailed. We had left those barbaric days of screaming women enduring the agony of labor and delivery.

Gradually, anesthesia became standard and as new anesthetic agents and techniques were developed they were quickly applied to the obstetrical patient. At the first whimper of distress obstetricians were ready with the bottles of pain relievers to inject or tanks of anesthetic gases to put an uncomfortable mamma-to-be out of her misery. The motives were honorable, but the results not always happy.

We now have thousands of pain relievers that can make labor and delivery more comfortable. Unfortunately, not one of them is completely safe for the about-to-be-born child. What's more, with most of them, the more pain relief you get the greater the risk to the infant.

In a sense you play a sort of trade-off game: mother's comfort for baby's safety.

The tendency of American physicians has been to opt in favor of the mother's comfort. The reasons aren't completely clear, but some possibilities come to mind. First, anesthesia was developed in this country; how natural for its use to become most widespread here. Second, medicine here is newer than in many of the European countries. After all, we've been around for two hundred years; they, for centuries. They've had the time to develop certain cultural traditions which never took hold in America, most notably home delivery and midwifery. Not that delivery at home by midwives is automatically or necessarily better than hospital delivery, but it does do one important thing: it increases the use of psychological support in childbirth and reduces the use of drugs.

Next, it's easier, faster and more compatible with a busy practice to simply give the delivering mother some drugs, rather than spend hours preparing her psychologically for the moment or standing by the bedside during labor and delivery, holding her hand.

Finally, the American practice of obstetrics has always focused more attention on the mother than on the baby. This, after all, is the patient that the doctor knows. If she has pain during labor and delivery, he has to watch her suffer: something no doctor enjoys. In addition, he'll have to answer to her. He may lose her as a patient and may lose her friends as well. The baby— well, he knows that the baby's there, but it's the mother who's his patient. If something bad happens to the baby, the obstetrician won't be pleased, but he also won't have to take care of him. That's the job of the pediatrician.

Make no mistake, obstetricians are well-intentioned. None of them wants to injure either the mother or the baby. They have simply been caught up in an evolutionary process, a natural flow of American obstetrics which has unconsciously but systematically emphasized maternal comfort at the expense of the baby's welfare.

To sort out the confusion about drugs versus "the natural way" in labor and delivery we'll divide the discussion into three easy-to-follow parts. First, what do drugs do to the baby and when and why are they dangerous? Here we'll consider all pain and anxiety relievers together. This includes injections in the region of the spinal cord—saddle blocks, epidurals, caudals and spinals—intravenous and intramuscular injections of pain relievers and sedatives, and the gaseous anesthetics that you inhale. Different drugs have different potencies and risks, but they have in common the tendency to depress the baby. Second, we will try to give you some practical advice so that you know how you can help insure that your baby is born in the safest possible fashion. If you do take some pain relievers, what should you take, when, and how much? Finally, a few words about each of the common obstetrical drugs so that you have a better idea which ones are the safest and why.

Effects of Drugs on the Emerging Baby

To offer you an overview, we've oversimplified this a bit. Some drugs are more potent and more risky than others. Some affect certain aspects of labor, delivery and newborn responses more than others. We'll straighten out some of these oversimplifications as we continue. First, we begin at the beginning: what happens in labor and delivery, and what effects do drugs in general have?

That time of life we call birth brings special challenges for this new child. The drug risks that were of serious concern earlier such as birth deformities, interference with proper growth, blocks in the normal smooth maturation of specialized organs are past. She is now fully formed and ready to take her place in the world.

To do this, she must be well-prepared to take over the life-supporting functions that her mother previously provided. Instead of getting oxygen and eliminating carbon dioxide wastes through her mother's bloodstream, her own lungs and circulatory system must do the job. Instead of relying on those nutrients that her mother provided through the placenta, she's now got to bring in her own food. Sure, her mother still has to provide her with the source—breast or bottle—but she must suck, swallow, digest and absorb those vital nutrients through her own digestive tract.

What's more, before the child can take over those self-supporting jobs, she's got to get out safely. That may seem easier to you than it really is. Millions of babies each year make the journey successfully, yet thousands of babies are also lost or permanently injured during birth. Getting out of the mother's body is a rough road; probably the toughest a human being ever faces.

Drugs before birth affect all aspects of this new independent life. They alter the birth process itself, and they alter vital centers in the baby's brain that control those life-giving functions of breathing and eating. How do they do this?

During labor the uterus begins to contract or squeeze down. As it does, the baby changes position and moves downward in the birth canal. At the same time, these contractions and this movement permit the cervix to dilate and widen so the baby can fit through and get out. The cervix (the lowest part of the uterus) is normally closed except for a narrow passageway, no wider than a small pencil. It must stretch little by little during labor until it is five inches or so across: big enough to let the baby out.

Two forces combine to push the baby downward and widen the cervical opening. The uterus itself squeezes tightly, forcing its living contents toward the exit. This squeezing or contraction is what you recognize as "labor pains." This comes about naturally and unconsciously. Even if you wanted to, you couldn't, by wishing or straining, make the uterus stop contracting.

The other force that helps you move toward that goal of expelling the baby is more under your control. You recall, if you have ever had a baby before, that your doctor or a nurse kept admonishing you to "push." You may have felt utterly exhausted and ready to give up yet that demand of "push," "push" kept calling for your last bit of energy. This active, conscious pushing contracts the muscles that line your belly wall, helping the forces of labor. It hastens the march of the baby downward and helps the cervix to widen.

Now it doesn't take much imagination to realize that drugs that dull your senses and make you relax might also affect the progress of labor. Many of the drugs that help take your pain away also keep the uterus from contracting as hard or as often. Others make you so groggy or weak that you can't possibly help things along by pushing.

In some unusual circumstances, slowing your labor down or giving you a needed rest period may be advantageous. You may have been straining for twenty hours, and labor may just not be going right. You and the baby, too, might need to relax and reenergize so you can start again, full of vigor. At times like those, drugs to help you rest may be essential for you and the baby.

Most often, however, labor will progress smoothly and well and should not be interrupted. Interrupting labor in midstream can be hazardous for the unborn child. For one thing, each uterine contraction may alter blood flow to the fetus and rob the baby of crucial oxygen (a few recent studies question this). Ideally the total number of contractions should be kept as few as possible so that these periods of vulnerability are minimized. Drugs, by making contractions weaker and less effective, can increase the number of uterine contractions needed to complete delivery.

Secondly, the longer labor goes on, the greater the chances for fetal complications. The umbilical cord can plunge outward and become squeezed, which stops the blood from flowing to the baby and threatens his life. The baby's head can pound excessively against the bones of his mother's pelvis, increasing risk of injury.

Finally, weakening of the propulsive forces may stop the baby's progress in a sort of no man's land in the middle of that bony outlet. The obstetrician may then be forced to use forceps, a kind of metal clamp, to pull the baby down. Forceps deliveries, though commonly done with no aftereffects, can be more dangerous than spontaneous self-propelled births. For all of these reasons, a basic philosophy in obstetrics is that labor and delivery should move along as rapidly and naturally as possible. Drugs, by slowing down both uterine contractions and maternal cooperation, can increase labor and delivery time and thereby jeopardize the emerging child.

Drugs may have other adverse effects, either while the baby is still inside his mother or at the moment he gets out. You may recall from Chapters 3 and 4 how markedly the unborn child depends upon her mother for supplying her life-giving oxygen and taking away poisonous waste products. How well mother performs this job depends upon how well she herself is breathing and how strong her blood pressure is. Many anesthetic agents can make mother breathe less effectively, and her blood oxygen level may fall. The mother normally takes in more oxygen than she needs and can do well even if she takes in somewhat less. The baby, on the other hand, lives in an environment of marginal oxygenation. She cannot afford to lose one bit of that precious life-giver. Small changes in the mother's respiration can produce a serious threat of suffocation for her baby.

The other factor that determines how well the baby gets the oxygen she needs is the quality of the blood flow from the mother to the uterus and placenta. This is determined, in part, by her blood pressure. Certain anesthetic agents can lower the mother's blood pressure. Once again, this minor reduction in blood pressure may mean very little to the mother, but the baby might not be so lucky. Her blood and oxygen needs are too delicately balanced to tolerate even relatively small changes in available blood from her mother. Injuries, particularly to brain centers, can result from oxygen deprivation.

Finally, all drugs used in labor and delivery get into the baby. Most of these sedatives and pain relievers are depressant drugs, and they can have the same effect upon the newborn, to a much greater degree. After all, what might have been a small amount of drug for a 120-pound mother, is a massive quantity for her seven-pound girl. All of the unwanted depressant effects of these drugs are magnified many times in this tiny child. How does this show up, and what does it mean?

In general, the more depressant, pain-relieving and sedative drugs that are given to the mother, the more depressed the baby is at birth. Degrees of depression may vary from a brief failure to take a breath or cry to complete depression and death. Fortunately, doctors know enough about the use of these drugs so that the latter disastrous effect is relatively rare. However, it is by no means unusual for newborns who were exposed to depressant drugs to remain blue for hours, to need some assistance with breathing for the first few minutes, to appear limp and weak and to suck poorly for the first few days of life. Although ironclad proof is lacking, common sense tells us that this just can't be good.

Most of us would also agree that the child who is vigorous and strong at birth is getting a better start on life. What about those infants who fall somewhere in between—not very perky, yet not totally out of it? Where do they stand? This is an important question since it applies to the majority of the infants whose mothers receive anesthesia for labor and delivery: in other words, a substantial fraction of our newborns.

Many doctors who deliver babies have adopted a rather strange philosophy about this group of youngsters. It's kind of an all-or-none theory. They make the assumption that the child is either normal or severely injured. They tell themselves and the mother that the baby who is lethargic, blue and fighting to breathe is just as well off as that vigorous, active newborn, as long as she starts breathing "soon enough." Reason tells us that this just can't be so. First of all, no one knows what "soon enough" really means. Secondly, brain injuries due to oxygen deprivation are not all-or-none. They span a continuous spectrum ranging from none at all to fatal. A brief look at simple brain physiology tells us why this is so.

Injuries that occur just before or at birth are generally due to hypoxia or insufficient oxygen. When the brain doesn't get enough oxygen for only a few minutes, cells begin to die. They are lost forever, as are the functions they were meant to serve. This loss of cells is not a sudden event but rather is gradual and progressive. Little, by little, as oxygen lack continues, more and more brain cells die. Those children who are born blue, breathe poorly or slowly and are severely depressed are far more likely to have some permanent injury than those who are alert and active at birth. The injury may not be gross or obvious. They may not be paralyzed or severely retarded, but some of their potential may be gone. Perhaps they'll develop what we call "hyperactivity." Or they may simply not be quite as intelligent or productive as they otherwise might have been.[1,5,8]

The easiest problems to identify and study are the grossly obvious and immediate signs. Almost all obstetrical educators agree that children born after their mothers are sedated are more depressed and less likely to breathe vigorously.[2,3] At the far extreme, the death rate is increased. In the United States we rank sixteenth among Western nations in perinatal mortality,[4] and one likely factor is our use of drugs in labor and delivery.

All of the countries with the lowest perinatal mortality, including Sweden, Finland, Japan, the Netherlands and Denmark, are far more judicious in their use of drugs. All of the countries with infant mortality rates comparable to ours, like Belgium, Israel, and England, have obstetrical practices that closely resemble ours. Moreover, as countries begin to "westernize"—that is, adopt American obstetrical anesthesia practices—their infant mortality rates rise concomitantly. The conclusion: we, the model for all the world, must be doing something wrong.

Of the babies that don't die shortly after birth—and this is the vast majority—there are still significant alterations in those who were exposed to lots of drugs before birth. They are more lethargic; they don't suck as well; they have greater weight losses in the early days after birth, and they are more likely to have abnormal EEG (brain wave) studies than infants who were not exposed to drugs prior to delivery.[5-7]

One study reviewed the later performance of children who were only very "slightly depressed" at birth by our standard measuring techniques. Those children were compared with children who at birth were more active, alert and vigorous. These "slightly depressed" children who would be considered "normal" by usual obstetrical standards were found to be less attentive at age one year than the ones who were most active at birth.[8] What this means in terms of lifelong performance is not clear, but perhaps even slight depression at birth, which physicians generally accept as "normal," may indeed lead to some permanent neurologic impairment.

The availability of potent anesthetic drugs has accelerated far faster than our understanding of their possible effects on the newborn child. Blue, depressed, gasping babies may come out all right in the end, but the automatic belief that they are bound to doesn't make much sense. It's time to revise our thinking, and new mothers may have to be the ones to get the ball rolling. A more sensible concept is that the more alert and vigorous the baby is from the moment of birth, the better his chances for optimal development.

In brief summary then, drugs alter the progress of labor and make delivery more difficult for the baby. They may lower the availability of oxygen by affecting the mother's respiration or blood pressure. Finally, they invade the body of the child, now nearly born, and alter his state of consciousness, strength and ability to breathe properly.

How To Improve the Safety of Labor and Delivery

There is no question that "natural" delivery techniques work. Until the late 1800s, all babies were born that way: there was no anesthesia. Even today, in most parts of the world, obstetrical anesthesia is used much less than here. No one is claiming that giving birth isn't painful. Labor and delivery can be excruciating. Various educational programs, some using special techniques such as hypnosis, have helped many women develop the attitude and frame of mind necessary to carry them through a drug-free labor and delivery.

We fully realize, however, that such programs don't work for everybody. People are different, as are birth experiences. Your labor may be exceedingly prolonged;

you may have an exceptional amount of pain; your ability to withstand pain may differ from your neighbor's. No need to be ashamed of that.

Finally, you may not be able to deliver in the standard manner, but may need a cesarean section, an operation that cuts your lower abdominal wall. We surely wouldn't recommend that you endure a surgical procedure without some pain relief. No—birth without drugs just isn't for everybody or every situation.

Quite likely, if you have never had a baby, you'll have no idea whether "natural childbirth" is for you or not. Even if you have, you might not know this time, since every delivery can be different. You might decide to take one of the several courses widely available to acquaint you with the "natural" techniques—we would urge this. Or you may decide that you can do without any drugs on your own. This may be all right for some of you, but in general the psychological support you get from the courses is quite helpful. It is often a useful substitute for medications.

The best-known "natural" childbirth methods are Lamaze and Bradley. If you live in a metropolitan area, you can find their numbers in the phone book. If you have problems deciding which method to choose, or, if you can't find the numbers, your obstetrician probably will be able to guide you. Enough women are interested in these methods today that obstetricians are familiar with them, whether they like them or not.

You may make the decision from the moment you become pregnant: "I'll try it without drugs," or you may decide, "I just know that's not for me." Finally, you may try to do it without drugs and then find that you need some relief once labor and delivery commences. If you do decide to take some pain relievers or an anesthetic, do so without feeling any guilt or shame. Everybody's needs are different. Moreover, if drugs are used carefully and properly the risk to your baby can be kept to a bare minimum. For those of you who will get some drugs (and after all, this will be the majority) we offer some facts about which are safest, and how and when they are best used.

Drugs for Labor and Delivery

The general rule is: don't take anything unless or until you absolutely need it. The reason for this is clear from our earlier discussion. The more drugs you take, the riskier it is for the baby, and the earlier you take them the more likely labor will be slowed. All too often, your doctor may order sedatives for many patients in labor, regardless of individual needs. This might even be done by phone without seeing you or determining how much discomfort you are actually having. For many physicians who deliver babies, drugs have become an automatic, almost reflex, response. "Mrs. Jones is here in earlier labor," says the nurse. "Give her ten milligrams of Valium," the doctor may reply.

We would caution you to take some responsibility. Have a discussion with your doctor long before your due date. Talk about labor and delivery drugs with him. Find out what types of drugs he normally uses and when. Let him know that you may want some relief, but that you want to decide when. You'll be the one to inform him or the nurse when you need some help. If someone wants to give you an injection when you're feeling reasonably comfortable, find out why. Is it something to calm you or help take the pain away? If so, perhaps you'd like to wait a little while.

Analgesics and Sedatives

This category includes a variety of tranquilizers, barbiturates, and narcotic drugs, like Demerol and morphine. These are used to help calm and relieve pain. They are given by injection, either through the intravenous line that may be dripping into your vein, or by a shot into your arm or buttock. These drugs are used quite commonly for women who are about to deliver. They can be a godsend of relief after hours of straining, hurting and fatigue.

Remember, however, that they are potent depressants and, the more relief you get, the greater the likelihood of depressing your baby. If you need them, ask for them, but only when absolutely necessary. In general, your doctor will try not to give these too near the moment of delivery. This will lessen the likelihood of significantly depressing your newborn. If you and the baby are followed closely, if your physician is attentive and careful with both dosages and timing of these drugs, they can be relatively safe.

Local Anesthetics

A variety of drugs, when they are injected around the nerve, have the property of stopping nerve messages. These are called "local anesthetics." You are likely to run into these near delivery, for they are the drugs the doctor may inject into your back or your vagina to produce a variety of nerve blocks. Spinal anesthesia, caudal anesthesia, epidural anesthesia, saddle blocks and pudendal blocks are names that may ring a bell. These have gained tremendous popularity in recent years, for in some ways they are both more effective and safer than other forms of anesthesia, but they are not without problems or totally devoid of hazard for the unborn child.

Certain of these blocks, particularly spinal anesthesia, may reduce the mother's blood pressure. This will probably affect her very little, but if you recall from our earlier discussion, the baby may not do well with even a small, or transient reduction of her blood supply.

They have other, potentially adverse effects. Many obstetricians believe that these drugs don't enter the baby's body. A recent report endorsed by the American College of Obstetrics and Gynecology made such a claim.[9] How nice it would be if this were true! Unfortunately, it is not. Local anesthetics are taken up by the mother's bloodstream and passed through the placenta to the fetus. As much as two-thirds of the maternal concentrations of these drugs can be found in the baby's blood after a short period of time.[10] The physical signs that the baby shows due to the presence of these local anesthetics include a drop in the heart rate while the child is still inside the mother and, occasionally, depression after birth.[11-13] Obstetricians and anesthesiologists can't let down their guard because of the misimpression that these drugs don't get into the baby. They do, and attentive observation and rapid treatment, if necessary, are vital.

Both of these problems—blood-pressure changes and newborn depression—can be managed fairly effectively if your doctor is attentive. After you have had a spinal anesthetic, for example, someone must stay with you constantly. At the first sign of blood-pressure change certain corrective measures can be taken quickly: increasing your intravenous fluids, raising your legs, and occasionally giving certain counteracting drugs. When the baby is born, your doctor must carefully examine the child to be sure that she is active and breathing well. If she is not, urgent corrective measures are in order.

Spinal and other regional anesthesias are useful adjuncts to modern obstetrics. Spinal anesthesia is particularly valuable if you need a cesarean section. Pain relief is complete, yet the effect on you and your child is not nearly as serious as a general anesthetic. There are still hazards, but if your doctor is careful and attentive, the risk to you and your unborn child can be minimized.

Inhalational Anesthesia

These drugs get into your body as you breathe them in. Certain inhalational anesthetics are useful for labor and delivery, and one deserves special mention.

Nitrous oxide, nicknamed "laughing gas," is commonly used by dentists in their offices. If the concentration of nitrous oxide is kept relatively low, it is quite safe for both mother and baby. It does get into the baby's system, mind you, but it is not as strong a respiratory depressant as many other drugs. It would be ideal except for one thing. It is not a potent pain reliever. However, it can take the edge off and may be all you need to get you through most of labor. Or, it may permit you to take less of those more potent drugs, thus decreasing the chances of newborn depression.

Other inhalational anesthetics such as halothane and cyclopropane are occasionally used, particularly for cesarean sections. They are strong drugs that can put you deeply asleep and totally eliminate pain. They are also potent depressants for the newborn. As many as 20 to 40 percent of infants who are exposed to these drugs before birth need some outside assistance to help them breathe after they are born.[2] Thus these drugs should only be used by highly skilled anesthesiologists who are prepared to ventilate the newborn artificially. It goes without saying that this is far from ideal. These drugs have a place in some situations (particularly in cesarean sections) in the hands of skilled physicians, but they pose a higher risk for the newborn than most of the other agents we have mentioned.

Summary

1. The use of sedatives and various pain relievers during labor and delivery is standard practice in this country. Often these drugs are used excessively with resulting injury, either obvious or subtle, to the newborn child.

2. No drugs are completely safe—all depress the baby to some extent. Furthermore, often the more relief you get, the more you risk your baby's welfare. An exception to this is the local anesthetics which may be given as a spinal, epidural, caudal, saddle or other types of blocks. These pose some hazard to the fetus but if monitoring is careful, the risk can be greatly reduced. They are generally less dangerous for the baby than injectable sedatives, narcotics and some of the gases that are inhaled.

3. If you can, have your baby without any drugs. Its the safest thing to do. For many of you, this simply isn't possible, so don't feel guilty. Simply try to get along with as little medication as you can. Discuss your concerns and wishes with your doctor be-

forehand. Don't accept a drug simply because it is the "routine" order from the doctor. You have the right to help decide that you need it.

4. If you do need drugs, some type of nerve block combined with small amounts of nitrous oxide and very little, if any, sedatives and narcotics, are your safest bet. However, exactly what you take must also be modified according to the experience of your doctor and the availability of other trained personnel.

Finally, if you do take some sort of pain-relieving medication, the likelihood is that your new baby will be just fine, providing your physician is skilled, judicious in his use of drugs, careful to monitor you and your baby closely and is ready to intervene quickly if trouble develops.

Section Four

INFECTIONS

XIV

German Measles (Rubella) and Other Viruses

Viruses are tiny germs, much smaller than any bacteria. They are peculiar creatures since, unlike bacteria, they can't live by themselves. Instead, they must invade the cells of an animal or plant, take over their machinery and make the captives do their bidding. Their bidding is always the same—make more viruses. They are, therefore, parasites that survive at the expense of others.

We can relate to bacteria, those one-celled living organisms who share our world. They are living independent creatures just as we are; most of them are harmless, and many are essential helpers of man. Viruses are rarely helpers; they are generally pests. They bring trouble ranging in intensity from a minor cold to fatal pneumonias or meningitis. Many of the viruses that bother adults can also affect the unborn child. Unfortunately, the growing embryo and fetus frequently suffer far more than their mothers.

Rubella (German Measles)

This is the classic example of how a virus, so inconsequential for the mother, can ravage a hapless growing infant. Rubella is commonly known as "the three-day measles," or "German measles."

It is unrelated to regular measles. When it strikes an

adult it may produce minor symptoms: a rash, a low-grade fever, a few aches, and swollen glands. It may be so mild that no symptoms whatsoever appear. The forming embryo is rarely so lucky.

When rubella strikes the mother in the first trimester, the growing infant runs a 50 percent chance of contracting the virus and having its development thrown into disarray.[1-5] The aftermath of congenital rubella may include malformations or improper development of almost every organ system. Eye malformations, heart defects, hearing impairment, stunting of brain growth, general growth failure, blood cell and clotting abnormalities, liver failure, pneumonia and weakened bones can all occur.[3-8] In 1964–1965 an epidemic of the disease in the United States left 30,000 maimed youngsters in its wake.

The end of the era of rubella-ravaged newborns is near. To bid it goodbye forever, you, a prospective mother, must do your part. We now have simple blood tests to tell whether or not you have ever had the disease. Remember, you may have had it, but it may have been so mild that you didn't know you had it. Or, you may think you've had it, because it resembles many other illnesses, when, in fact you never did.

If the blood test shows that you have had the disease, you and your baby are safe. You can't get it again. If the test is negative, we now have an immunizing vaccine that will protect you and your baby. This vaccine is now routinely given to preschool youngsters to keep them from contracting rubella. Not that it's dangerous for them, but we don't want them to carry it home to their expectant mothers.

Long before you contemplate becoming pregnant you must have a rubella test. If the test shows that you are vulnerable, you must be vaccinated. One very strong caution: vaccinations can never be given to women who are pregnant, might be pregnant or could become pregnant in the next three months. You see, the vaccine itself can infect the growing baby and produce the same congenital injuries as the natural viral infection.

If you do get vaccinated by mistake while you are

pregnant, or become pregnant within three months after vaccination, there is a small chance that your child will contract congenital rubella. Fortunately, that chance is far, far less than if you actually got German measles itself. Many women who were inadvertently vaccinated during pregnancy have given birth to normal youngsters. An unlucky few, however, do have deformed babies. If you are vaccinated near the beginning of pregnancy, abortion is usually advised just to be safe. If your personal beliefs eliminate abortion as a possible solution, chances are fairly good that things will turn out all right.[9,10]

If you have just become pregnant, and had a rubella test which proved negative, you could have a problem. You need repeated tests to be sure that you don't contract the illness during those first critical months of pregnancy. If the test never becomes positive, there's nothing to worry about. Your baby is safe. If it does, you face a very serious personal decision. Do you interrupt the pregnancy with an abortion or do you take your chances and have the child? That, of course, is a decision only you can make. As we indicated, the chances are not in your favor. There is a 50–50 chance that the child will be malformed or defective.[1-4]

Influenza ("Flu")

True influenza can pose a serious threat to the unborn child. Before you get too concerned, however, let's clarify one thing. The term "flu" is overused and misused by laymen and physicians alike. It has come to mean everything from a mild stomach upset to diarrhea to a slight cold. For some reason these have all been dubbed "flu" even though, in general, they are due to other types of milder viral infections. True flu or influenza is an epidemic disease that strikes large numbers of people at once. It is not a mild illness: high fevers, shaking chills, severe cough, muscle aches and physical prostration are the characteristic signs of true influenza. Influenza can be a fatal disease to the mother as well as to the unborn child. Millions died in the great world-wide epidemic of 1918. Many thousands died in the Asian flu pandemic of 1957.

If you contract true influenza while you are pregnant, chances are approximately 50–50 that you will lose the baby. More often than not, miscarriages or stillbirths occur.[8,11,12] If this does not happen and your pregnancy continues, the likelihood is that the baby will not be injured. While there is a higher incidence of brain injuries in children exposed to influenza while inside their mothers, the incidence is fairly low.[7,8]

Because influenza can be so devastating to a pregnancy, and because the vaccines to prevent it are relatively safe for the unborn child, most officials recommend vaccinating pregnant women when an epidemic is expected. Better to be vaccinated before you become pregnant, but if you didn't make it, you might consider getting the vaccine during your pregnancy. One note of caution: different vaccines are used against different forms of influenza, and they may vary in nature. Check with your doctor to be sure that vaccination of pregnant women with the vaccine currently in use is advised. The Center for Disease Control and the Food and Drug Administration will generally make those recommendations available to the practicing physician.

The Common Cold

The common cold is the most prevalent and probably the most irksome of all viral illnesses. Unlike measles, mumps, chicken pox or rubella, which attack only once and leave us immune and protected forever, colds are far more tricky. Many different types of viruses may give us the runny, sniffly nose that we recognize as "a cold." That is the main reason we can get colds over and over again—the attacking army is forever changing, leaving us open to repeated assaults.

Your colds don't bother the unborn child, which is lucky, since probably most women catch a cold during pregnancy. If you get one, sniffle away and don't let it bother you. Avoid taking excessive aspirin or cold remedies, as you were warned in Chapters 9 and 10.

Measles

Measles is another of the many viral diseases that is gradually being relegated to the history books. Most adults have been exposed or have actually had the disease; thus they have protecting antibodies. Most children are now being immunized with vaccines developed in the past few years; thus they won't get it. More important, particularly when you are pregnant, they won't bring it home to you. The likelihood is, therefore, that either you are not susceptible or you won't be exposed, or both.

That's fortunate, since measles is a serious disease when you are pregnant. Your unborn child is seriously threatened if you get measles. Certain developmental abnormalities, particularly of the brain, can occur.[6,7] More often, however, miscarriage or stillbirth is the sad result of measles during pregnancy.[6,13]

Hepatitis

Infection of the liver by the hepatitis viruses can seriously complicate a pregnancy. The child can come out unscathed, but chances of premature delivery, low birth weight and liver involvement of the baby himself are approximately 25 percent.[6,7] Chances are also frighteningly high that the child will die shortly after birth. The death rate is about 22 percent.[14] As with all other viral infections, there is no good treatment or cure. The only hope is to minimize exposure. Using dirty hypodermic needles, sharing others' drinks, eating raw shellfish are some of the common ways that the hepatitis viruses are transmitted.

Mumps

Like measles, mumps is fading rapidly from the medical picture. Their illness or exposure to it in childhood and new vaccines make it unlikely that many pregnant women will get this disease. Mumps is generally a relatively mild illness, although it does occasionally lead to some complications in infected adults. If the pregnant woman contracts the disease during the first trimester chances are about one in four that she will lose the baby.[7] The other 75 percent generally do well, and there is no good evidence that links any fetal deformities to prenatal exposure to mumps. Fetuses exposed after the first trimester have a good likelihood of successfully growing, developing and reaching the outside world as healthy human beings.

Herpes Simplex

This is a viral infection that deserves very special mention. Unlike mumps, measles and some of the other viral illnesses that are on their way out, herpes is on the upswing. What's more, it poses a very serious threat to the unborn child. Common herpes infections are the familiar "fever blisters" or "cold sores" that you get in and around your mouth. The more serious form of the infection, at least for the unborn child, is venereal herpes which produces similar blister-like lesions on the genital area and is transmitted by sexual contact. It is most important that you have regular gynecological checkups during pregnancy to look for any signs of herpes infection. It may be very mild, unnoticeable and harmless for you, but it can be quite dangerous to the unborn child.

No one knows how frequently the unborn child is infected when his mother has a herpes infection. We do know that the virus is transmitted to the baby both through the placenta and through direct contact when the newborn traverses the birth canal.[3,4,6,7] Herpes infections of the newborn are catastrophic. They spread like wildfire throughout his entire body, involving almost every organ, and the mortality rate of infected newborns is approximately 70 percent.[15]

Summary

This covers only a few of the very common viral infections to which pregnant women may be exposed.

Some of them are harmless to the unborn child, others are catastrophic. Birth defects, and death before or shortly after birth are some of the possible consequences when these viral infections invade the tissues of the growing child. Some of them can be prevented by proper screening and immunization before you become pregnant: measles, rubella (German measles), mumps and influenza are examples.

Others can be controlled only by reducing your exposure: the risk of contracting herpes is lessened if you minimize the number of different sexual encounters. Hepatitis is less likely to strike if you avoid contact with known carriers, don't use dirty hypodermic needles, avoid raw shellfish and don't share other people's glasses or silverware. The common cold won't hit as often if you avoid crowds and direct contact with people who have colds. Since most viral infections can't be treated effectively, you owe it to yourself and your unborn child to do your best to stay healthy.

XV

Infections Caused by Bacteria

A discussion of infections wouldn't be complete without casting at least a passing glance at bacteria, oldest known members of the germ world. Bacteria are one-celled plants that live around and within us in quantities so large that our minds can't comprehend them. They are everywhere: in the air, the soil, the food we eat and in our own bodies.

Yes, right inside us. Hundreds of species of bacteria live in our mouths and intestinal tracts. We give them a place to live and they pay for their room and board by helping us to digest our food, providing us with certain vitamins and helping our bowels to function smoothly and efficiently.

We get along well as long as they stay where they belong. Many of those bacteria can be quite harmful to their human hosts if they escape from their normal confines. We can become very sick if they invade our lungs, our peritoneal (abdominal) cavities, our bladder and kidneys, our brains or our bloodstreams.

When bacteria find their way into places where they aren't welcome we call this a "bacterial infection." A common throat infection, "strep throat" is caused by a particular bacterium which doesn't normally belong there. That bacterium is called *Streptococcus,* hence the familiar nickname. The red streaks that can course up your arm or leg after you've been cut or had a puncture wound (perhaps you've called this "blood poisoning") is a *Streptococcus* infection at another location.

Different types of bacteria can cause infections of the lungs (pneumonia); infections of the spinal cord and brain (meningitis); infections of the heart valves (endocarditis); infections of the abdominal lining (peritonitis); infections of the kidneys (pyelonephritis); infections that are transmitted through sexual contact (venereal diseases), and so on.

When bacteria infect adults they may cause a wide variety of derangements. However, they usually are harmless to the unborn child. Unlike viruses, which almost invariably enter the fetal tissues, bacteria that infect the mother rarely do.

There are only a few instances when a mother's bacterial infection can be detrimental to the unborn child. The first instance is when the pregnant woman is seriously or deathly ill. Her inability to eat, her high fever —if these are prolonged or extreme—can lead to fetal death and miscarriage. Scarlet fever, typhoid fever, cholera and a number of other bacterial illnesses that you are unlikely to contract may end this way.

The more common bacterial diseases, including strep throat, kidney infection, bladder infection and pneumonia, are more likely to leave behind a healthy, living baby, assuming that you don't become unusually ill, are treated in a timely manner and respond well to the chosen drugs.

The second instance when a mother's bacterial infection can be injurious to the unborn child is in the uncommon case when the bacteria spreads to the fetus through the placenta. Tuberculosis occasionally does. When it does, the mother is usually deathly ill herself with so-called "military tuberculosis," and often both she and her baby die. Syphilis is the other common bacterial infection which invades the fetal tissues directly. This bug is particularly sneaky, since the mother will frequently be symptom-free at a time when her unborn child is being engulfed by life-threatening bacteria. We discussed the problems of congenital syphilis, its prevention, diagnosis and treatment in Chapter 12.

Finally, bacterial infections can be transmitted from

mother to newborn at the time of delivery or shortly before. Gonorrhea is one that we considered in Chapter 13. Others may be caused by bacteria that aren't even foreign to the mother. Normal bacterial residents of the vagina can gain access to the baby after the amniotic sac (water bag) breaks. The longer delivery is delayed after rupture of the sac, the greater is the opportunity for the unborn child to become infected with his mother's vaginal bacteria. He may be born with pneumonia, skin infections, or even fatal bacterial infections of the bloodstream. Fortunately, delivery normally follows soon after the sac ruptures, but not always. To minimize risk of this kind of infection, if your amniotic sac breaks before labor begins, have your doctor examine you—don't wait until the contractions start.

Summary

A mother's bacterial infections are generally less serious for the unborn child than are her viral infections. Strep throat, bladder infections, kidney infections and pneumonias are usually bacterial. Most of them, if treated promptly, won't hurt the baby.

There are a few instances when bacterial infections can pose a serious threat: first, if you are extremely ill; second, if you are infected by one of those rare bacteria that pass directly into the baby's body—the bacteria that cause tuberculosis and syphilis are the best known; third, if your baby picks up an infection after your membranes rupture or on his way out—gonorrhea is of greatest concern in this instance.

XVI

Cats and Raw Meat

Have we captured your attention with the title of this chapter? We hope so, for this fascinating tale has serious implications for your unborn child.

Since this isn't a mystery novel, let's give away the end of the story. What is the connection between cats and raw (or rare) meat?

Both cats and various food animals often are carriers of a tiny infectious organism known as *toxoplasma*. Toxoplasma are one-celled creatures, like bacteria. But unlike bacteria, they have certain characteristics that make them animals rather than plants. Officially they fall, along with amoeba and trichomonas, in that group of smallest living animals known as "protozoa."

These bugs are amazingly prevalent. Somewhere between 10 and 85 percent of American adults are invaded one time or another.[1-8] This doesn't mean that as many actually get sick, for often protozoa creep unnoticed into the adult body. The way we detect past exposure is by measuring antibodies, or special disease-fighting molecules made by the body, which are specifically directed against the toxoplasma. Indications are that as many as 50 million American adults carry such antibodies.

Like rubella and some of the other mild illnesses that we suffer, toxoplasmosis often comes and goes without really bothering us. Occasionally a rash, swollen glands, painful joints and muscles and even pneumonia may announce the presence of this uninvited guest, but more often than not the silent creature passes through unnoticed.

Mama may escape unscathed; the unborn child is rarely so lucky. When the bugs invade the mother, they generally pass directly into the unborn child. The forming infant lies defenseless—he can't make the antibodies or muster the bodily protection that his mother can.

The organs most commonly affected by the invading toxoplasma protozoa are the brain, the eye and the liver. Birth defects may include fatal liver or brain failure; mental retardation; hydrocephalus, commonly known as "water on the brain"; cerebral palsy; seizures or convulsions, and—very commonly—destruction of the retina with resulting blindness. Sounds bleak? For those who are unaware of the danger it may be. The incidence is shockingly high. For those who take some simple precautions, the chances of giving birth to an infected child are quite low.

To help you understand why you've got to do your part, here are a few concrete numbers for you to grasp. The estimated infection rate in this country is approximately one in every 3,000 pregnancies.[1,3] If you do contract an infection, there is approximately a 40 percent chance that your unborn child will become infected. This means that one in every thousand babies or 3,000 babies in the United States per year are born with the disease.[3] Of the children born with the infection, about 5 to 10 percent will die shortly after birth; 10 percent will have severe brain and/or eye damage; 10 to 13 percent will have moderately severe to severe visual handicaps, and the other 60 to 70 percent will have no symptoms at first, but run a high risk of developing serious visual problems as children or young adults.[3-5] If you add these percentages up, anywhere from 75 to 98 percent of the children born with the infection will have some serious handicap. The numbers of babies at risk and the severe consequences of the infection make toxoplasmosis a more serious public health problem today than either rubella or phenylketonuria; yet these latter diseases enjoy the spotlight of public attention, while toxoplasmosis is buried in obscurity.

Why are we giving you these scary statistics? Why

do we raise the specter of an illness that you have never even heard of? The reason: to clue you in about a potential health hazard which is probably new to you; not at all esoteric, but rather common, and, most important of all, *avoidable* if you know what to do about it.

After years of probing investigation that would be the envy of Sherlock Holmes, scientists have found some important answers. They have learned that members of the cat family, including the common house cat, as well as wild relatives like leopards, ocelots, cougars and bobcats, are nature's primary carriers of toxoplasma.[8] Other animals, including ones that we normally eat, such as pigs, cattle and sheep, and those that cats may eat, like mice and rats, may also carry the bug. However, only cats are what parasitologists call the "final host." By that we mean that the infectious organism can fully reproduce, complete a sexual cycle and make new eggs within the intestinal tract of the cat.[8] Those other animal hosts can carry eggs and cysts than can infect a predator that eats them, but they do not provide a suitable site for multiplication of toxoplasma organisms; only the cats do that.

The important questions for you, if you are a cat owner, are, "How does my cat become infected, and how might he give that infection to me?" Domestic cats normally get the infection by eating a rodent that is carrying eggs or cysts. You may think to yourself, "My cat never eats any mice or rats, so I have nothing to worry about." You might be right, but you can't be sure.

Mice and rats abound in cities, the countryside, and in our homes. You may never see them, but they are there, and you can be sure that your cat will be the first to find them. So even if you think that dear little Felix has never done anything as repulsive as eating a mouse or rat, don't count on it. If you live in a sixteenth-story apartment, and Felix has never gone outside since birth, and you feed him only canned cat food, then, chances are smaller that he's been infected. However, you still can't be sure, since mice can reach the most unexpected places. The likelihood is that your cat lies between these extremes. You may never have seen him eating a mouse, but you have probably let him run outside unattended. If that's your situation, chances are pretty good that your cat carries toxoplasmosis.

To protect your unborn child, you must assume that your cat harbors the bug and that he can pass it on to you if you aren't careful. What do you do? You were looking for an excuse to be free of that annoying cat anyway—you've found a great one. The best way to protect your baby is to be cat-free. But if you are fond of your cat, you don't have to send him away for nine months to be relatively safe.

Your cat passes the organisms along through his feces. They end up in the litter box, the soil outside, and your children's sandboxes, depending upon where he goes and where he tramples with his contaminated feet. Clearly, the greatest risk to you comes from the contaminated litter box. There millions of microscopic bugs are likely to reside. To protect your unborn child, don't empty your cat's litter box at any time while you are pregnant. Avoid, as much as possible, coming in contact with your pet's waste. Wash your hands thoroughly with soap and water after you have handled the animal, neatened up his sleeping blanket or put his toys away. In short, be on your guard. Be sure that your hands don't move from your cat, his feces or anywhere that he might have tracked microscopic waste particles, to your mouth, until you have thoroughly scrubbed them.

Just a brief aside for those of you who have a dog rather than a cat and are wondering about him. At the risk of alienating cat lovers everywhere, we must tell you the facts: dogs aren't a problem. They don't carry the toxoplasmosis organism or any common disease that may infect your unborn child.

Many of you don't have a cat and may feel that this doesn't concern you. Well, it does. This is where the raw (or rare) meat part comes in. We mentioned earlier that our food animals can carry eggs and cysts of the toxoplasma protozoa. They pick these up from the soil, and from the grasses they eat. Among our staple meats, pork and mutton are most commonly infected; beef more rarely. To avoid picking up the bug and passing it to your unborn child, all your meat should be well-cooked—heat kills the infecting bugs. No more nibbling on that raw hamburger meat. No more rare steaks until those nine months are over.

Summary

1. You may never have heard of toxoplasmosis, an illness caused by a small protozoan parasite, but it is a common and serious problem for the unborn child. Approximately 3,000 babies per year in the United States are born with this disease. Results include severe brain and liver injuries, and damage to the seeing mechanism of the eye with resulting blindness.
2. The main carriers of the disease are house cats and rare or raw meats. You can nearly eliminate the danger to your unborn child by taking a few simple steps.
   A. Don't empty your cat's litter box while you are pregnant. Let someone else do it. Wash your hands thoroughly after you have handled your cat or any of his items, particularly before you eat.
   B. Never eat raw or rare meats. Make sure that the meat you eat is well done.

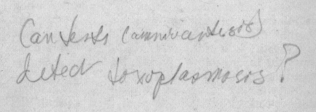

Section Five

THINGS IN YOUR ENVIRONMENT

XVII

Chemicals in
Common Foods

Food additives and accidental chemical intruders are routinely present in our daily diets. Like automobiles, television and Sunday football games, they are part of today's life. Emulsifiers, "flavor enhancers," artificial colors, preservatives and artificial sweeteners are added intentionally. Insecticides, herbicides, fertilizers, mercury, arsenic and industrial wastes steal in uninvited.

Food cultists have lumped all of these chemicals collectively under the label of "unnatural." They believe that so-called "organically" grown produce contains powers far beyond those of mortal vegetables. They would ban chemical fertilizers and insecticides, and as a result, this "organically grown" produce is often puny and infected.

Alarmists condemn all so-called "unnatural" food additives like citrate and glutamate. They fail to realize that these chemicals are common biochemicals which are produced in large quantities by our very own bodies. They recoil at the thought of preservatives like nitrates being added to meats—hot dogs, bacon, chopped meat, ham—when, in fact, many vegetables, including spinach, beets, radishes, celery, and cabbage contain hundreds of times as much. They call for the elimination of all man-made materials from our food supply, which means that fertilizers, insecticides, preservatives, colors and sweeteners would all have to go. The motive, to protect us food consumers, is well-intentioned but their notions are often ill founded.

Consumer protection is something we all believe in and strive to achieve. After all, isn't that the purpose of this book? But demands, blanket prohibitions, and uninformed recommendations are not the answer. Understanding the issues and applying benefit-risk concepts are vital to decision-making in matters that affect our well-being.

On the other side of the fence are the commercial food producers. They would like us to believe that "not known to be dangerous" means the same thing as "safe." They insist that if we cannot be certain of the danger of a potential food additive, then restricting its use is unjustified. They would like us to accord the same constitutional rights to chemicals that we American citizens enjoy—"innocent until proven guilty." This is no more correct than sweeping prohibitions. Chemical food additives and contaminants are by no means innocent until proven guilty.

Remarkably, food producers claim that consumer demands are their motivating force. People want artificial coloring, flavor enhancers, emulsifiers, and artificial sweeteners. Industry would have us believe that producers aren't at fault for adulterating our food: we consumers are. Madison Avenue advertising isn't designed to sell products, it's designed to give us what we want. Are we so naive as to believe that?

Somewhere between these two extremes rational answers can be found. You probably have some concerns about some of those chemicals in your foods, and you may worry about their potential effects on your unborn child. Well, there is some cause for concern and for exercising intelligent judgment in your food shopping. But don't let the hullabaloo about the nasty things you're eating scare you to death or make you a foodophobic. Let's put some things into proper perspective so you can eat well with confidence.

First, a little philosophy about some of those chemicals that have entered our food supply. Then a bit of advice for you.

Chemical fertilizers are a modern necessity. We depend for our food on the two percent of our people who till the soil and raise our crops. They can't supply all of us without using chemical fertilizers. Recent publicity has lauded the alleged superiority of "organic" fertilizers over their chemical counterparts, but this claim simply isn't true. Plants grown in chemical fertilizers aren't one bit different from those grown "organically." Americans have been duped into believing that there is a difference between "organic" and chemical fertilizers and the booming "organic" and "natural" food industries are the beneficiaries of this grand hoax. So put to rest any concerns you might have about chemical fertilizers: they are important, and they are safe.

Insecticides and some herbicides are also necessary. Without them farmers can't grow crops efficiently. If you have ever had a fruit tree in your back yard you know what we mean. Before you can collect the first harvest the fruit has been riddled by pests, unless, of course, you've sprayed them.

Take a look at the fruits and vegetables in the "natural" food markets—it's likely that those insects that have beaten you to the fruits and vegetables carry more disease than minute remnants of insecticides could ever bring. Not that we want insecticides or herbicides in our foods: they're not good for us or our unborn children either. However, they are the lesser of two evils. The solution isn't to eliminate them, because that can't be done. It's to scrub and wash your fresh produce thoroughly before you eat it.

Chemical preservatives are, to some extent, a necessary byproduct of our modern urbanized lifestyles. It may take days or weeks for foods to move from the farms or the slaughterhouses into your refrigerator. Without preservatives many would spoil. Then the majority of us city folk would end up hungry from food shortages or deathly ill from eating rotten, bacteria-laden meats and produce.

Keep in mind also the new lifestyle of many of today's women. Many of you work, and very few want to spend an hour or two every day food shopping, as your grandmother did. For the convenience of once-a-week food shopping, you accept long-lasting canned and preserved foods.

Are preserved foods safe? Well, we're not certain, but to date they seem to pose slight if any risk to you and your unborn child. It's important to point out here that many preservatives are actually "natural" chemicals that abound in our fruits, vegetables and grains. They've merely been adapted for use as preservatives.

On the one hand, we accept fertilizers, insecticides, and some preservatives as essential to modern healthful food production. But artificial flavors, colors, sweeteners, flavor enhancers, emulsifiers and other agents that change the texture and quality of foods are another matter entirely.

They are in our foods for one purpose only—to market products. Of course, we've gotten used to them and might be temporarily unhappy if we lost them. When we analyze why, it becomes clear that we've been sold a bill of goods.

Through fancy and convincing marketing techniques, manufacturers and distributors have made our mouths water over red, not naturally brownish meats; brightly colored beverages; and rainbow candies. Convenience desserts that whip up into frothy smooth peaks of "goodness" in only minutes have moved from the realm of laboratory curiosities into everyday dietary staples. Artificial sweetners, once touted as medicines for use by diabetics, are now consumed at the rate of thousands of tons per year.

Critical observers are rightly concerned. Their reasons: for one thing, these man-made chemicals are just window dressing. They have little known benefit except to sell foods. Secondly, are they harmful? So far we don't know, but remember that a number of them, used for years with confidence, have fallen into disrepute and have been removed from the marketplace.

Cyclamates and, more recently, saccharine, types of artificial sweeteners, and red number two food dye, formerly the most common red coloring used, are well-known examples. We ate them for years before they were discovered to cause cancers in experimental animals. The alarm rang out and off the market they came. "Oops!" said the FDA. "Maybe they're not so good for us after all."

Where does this leave you, the pregnant woman, concerned about the chemicals you may be eating? Should you be afraid to touch anything but home-grown produce, chickens and pigs you slaughter from your own backyards and milk you get from your faithful cow? Of course not! You have to eat a well-balanced, store-bought diet, unless you're among the two percent or so of our citizens who wake up to the crowing of your own roosters. Here are some practical recommendations.

The concept of "organically" grown foods is admir-able, but impractical. Don't worry about chemical ferti-lizers and insecticides. Buy plump, juicy and worm-free fruits and vegetables (you're less likely to find them in the "natural" foodstores than in your neighborhood supermarket). Scrub them well with soap and water to remove any possible trace of insecticides. Rinsing them lightly isn't good enough.

None of the common preservatives is now known or suspected of being hazardous to the unborn child. If you can, increase your intake of fresh, unpreserved foods, but don't turn your life upside down running away from all preservatives. Some are necessary and unavoidable. In many cases the foods are much safer with than without preservatives. Furthermore, many common preservatives are also common, natural chemi-cals. Nitrates, as mentioned earlier, and citric acid, the substance that gives citrus fruits their sour taste, are common preservatives. Ascorbic acid, vitamin C, is used for its antioxidant preservative qualities. Acetic acid (vinegar), lactic acid (a common plant and ani-mal chemical), calcium phosphate (a normal constitu-ent of our own bodies), are a few other commonly used preservatives.

Some preservatives are derived from petroleum and other non-edible sources. These include Benzoic acid,

BHA and BHT. These aren't natural and we may someday learn that they aren't healthful, but for now they are indispensable.

Artificial colors and sweeteners may not harm your unborn child. In fact, it's likely that they won't, but we aren't truly sure how safe they are. Furthermore, since you should be able to reduce your consumption of these with simple changes in your food-buying habits, we recommend that you try to keep these out of your grocery carts. Read labels. Substitute more natural foods for highly processed or fully manufactured ones. For example, make your own fresh lemonade or use bottled whole fruit juices instead of those powdered or canned drinks and sodas.

Use naturally sweetened desserts and beverages rather than those containing artificial sweeteners. Recall from Chapter 6 that you need the calories that sugar provides when you are pregnant. Saccharin, now being removed from the market, has no caloric value. What's more, it readily enters fetal tissues and may accumulate in high concentration in some of them. Does it hurt the baby? No one knows. But why take the chance? Every rule of biochemistry and common sense tells us that natural sugars must be safer than saccharin—a chemical that does not exist in nature.

Now there may be a few of you who should be using artificial sweeteners for sound medical reasons. If you are diabetic, have gained excessive weight or had a complication of pregnancy from those extra pounds, your doctor may want you to avoid sugar. If so, artificial sweeteners may be in order. For most of you, however, who have simply adopted artificial sweeteners as a way of life because you have a weight problem, or because of those convincing TV ads, think again. Do you really want to swallow loads of unnecessary, unnatural chemicals that end up in your baby's body?

Summary

1. Blanket bans to keep all man-made substances out of the food supply and food production are impractical and unnecesary.

2. Chemical fertilizers, insecticides and herbicides are essential to modern food production.
3. Pick store-bought produce for size and visual quality. Then scrub your produce well before serving it to yourself and your family.
4. Some chemical preservatives are also unavoidable. Some, like nitrates, are far more prevalent in certain natural vegetables than they are in preserved foods. Others, like citrate, are natural chemicals that are produced by our own bodies and help them run properly. As much as you can, eat unpreserved fresh foods, but you can eat preserved foods on occasion with relative assurance that they won't harm your unborn child.
5. Minimize your intake of artificially colored foods and avoid artificial sweeteners unless they are specifically ordered by your doctor. Sugar and other natural sweeteners are readily available.

XVIII

X Ray and Sonography

Ever since the days of Flash Gordon and his ray gun, people have worried about radiation. They might not have known why, or even what it was, but they knew it was scary. That gut feeling is true. Radiation can be very dangerous. However, if used carefully and properly it can also be a great ally; a friend that modern man can't afford to lose.

Radiation is energy that travels through the air. It takes many different forms and is carried in many different ways. Nuclear energy relies on atomic and smaller-than-atomic particles to distribute its energy. X rays, another form of radiation, are not particles but are electromagnetic waves, like light waves. They differ from visible light only in that they have shorter wavelengths that make them able to penetrate dense objects. This is the property that makes them so useful: they can go through our bodies and help us see what's inside. This same characteristic of short wavelength also gives them energy and the ability to destroy tissues. This is what makes X rays dangerous.

When Wilhelm Konrad Roentgen (1845–1923) took the first X-ray picture in 1895, the technique was an instant success. It became both a tool for medical advances and a toy, a curiosity. People were fascinated by this magical device that could see through things. Little did they know that this seemingly harmless machine, not much different outwardly from a light bulb, was more powerful and more lethal than anything man had ever known before.

It took years before the destructive powers of X rays were finally recognized. Thousands of early radiologists and non-medical dabblers who used these machines died. No one suspected that X rays were harmful, and skin cancers became common, since protective lead gloves and aprons were never worn. Leukemias and other cancers also took their toll of early X-ray specialists. Roentgen himself fell victim to his own invention, a real-life Doctor Frankenstein. The monster that he created would be a godsend for those in need; but until it could be controlled, it annihilated those who got in its way, including its own creator.

After many years the hazards of X rays became apparent; yet years passed before medical and federal regulatory agencies moved to control them. You may recall, not very long ago, when every neighborhood shoe store boasted an X-ray machine. What an after-the-movie treat, on Saturday afternoons, for kids to crowd into the store and watch each other's bones wiggle inside their shoes! It was fun all right, but it also bombarded those feet, and who knows what other parts of the body, with dangerous X-ray beams. At last, someone said, "Hey! What is this! Why have we permitted this uncontrolled toying with X-ray machines for all these years?" Finally they were removed.

X rays were used indiscriminately for medical reasons, too. Thousands of 20- and 30-year-olds today have suffered the delayed consequences of childhood X-ray treatment. Cancers of the thyroid and lymph glands are springing up around the world. The cause: X-ray irradiation 20 or more years ago, often to treat tonsillitis.

Many of these unnecessary and dangerous applications of X-ray techniques have fallen into disfavor. Still, even today, X rays are overused. You may be aware of the current controversy surrounding mammography. Some scientists are concerned that these routine annual X-ray examinations for breast cancer may actually produce more cancers than they uncover. Many believe that only those above a certain age who are most likely to harbor a hidden cancer should be exposed to the radiation of mammograms. They reason that young women, age 30 or so, probably shouldn't have X rays shot into their breasts year after year for the next three decades.

X rays, of course, can be indispensable to modern medical diagnosis and treatment. The broken bone, the pneumonia in your lung, the chicken bone that stuck in your throat, the ulcer in your stomach and thousands of other serious problems would be hidden from view if it weren't for the miracle of X rays. They are great friends when we need them, but when they are misused or used unnecessarily they turn against us. This is most definitely true in the case of the pregnant woman and her unborn child.

Radiation of any form can disrupt normal cell mechanisms and throw cells and tissues into disarray. When we use X rays to treat cancers, that's the desired effect: disturb those cancer cells and make them die. But if radiation reaches the vulnerable tissues of the unborn child, the effects may not be so desirable. The development of a particular organ or structure might be upset, resulting in a congenital deformity or malformation. Cells may be altered so that sooner or later they grow out of control—this is what we know as cancer. Finally, the genes of the sperm and ovum might be altered. This might lead to mutations which affect future generations—the offspring of those exposed unborn children.

Birth defects, cancers and mutations producing permanent genetic changes that are passed down for generations can all be produced by X rays and other forms of radiation in laboratory animals. Of greatest concern to you: how dangerous are the more or less routine X-ray pictures that you might have taken in your doctor's office or a hospital?

The clearest answer to that question has come from a living laboratory that we all regret and hope to never see again: the Hiroshima and Nagasaki bomb sites. Adults, children and unborn children who survived the nearby atomic blasts, have been observed ever since.

We've learned that radiation exposure of that intensity can be disastrous for the unborn child, and that the type and extent of injury is closely related to the distance of the mother from the bomb site—in other words, the radiation dosage.

Many fetuses died, pariculary those that received a high radiation dose. Many of the survivors were born with congenital defects, including microcephaly, retardation, and eye deformities.[1-3] A shocking number of the seemingly normal newborns developed cancers later in life—many during their childhood years. The most common cancers involved the lymph nodes and the blood-forming organs—leukemias—but others occurred as well.[1,2]

It's still too early to tell whether permanent genetic mutations have occurred that will affect later generations. There is one suspicious sign that prenatal exposure to radiation did produce some alterations in the productive genes of exposed fetuses. The normal ratio of 1.2 girls to 1 boy seems to be reversed in the offspring of today's Japanese adults who were exposed before birth.[4] This, in itself, may not seem like a serious problem, but it may be the first warning of worse things to come. After all, if the genetic machinery of these fetuses was disturbed so that the sex of the progeny was affected, there might be more serious genetic injuries which will crop up later.

You may wonder what this all has to do with you. After all, you hope you won't find yourself in an atomic blast. The answer is that radiation exposure of all types, from the everyday X ray to a major atomic blast, shares certain destructive characteristics. The amount of destruction and the degree of risk is proportional to the magnitude of radiation exposure.

The two modern situations which come closest in destructive quality (though they are still considerably less) to those atomic blasts are fallout from nuclear tests and therapeutic radiation. Some studies have identified higher incidences of congenital defects in children born hundreds of miles from nuclear test sites. It would appear that even relatively low levels of nuclear fallout can jeopardize the growing fetus.[5]

X-Ray Therapy

Therapeutic radiation (high-energy radiation such as cobalt, radium, etc.) is used to treat cancers. Women who develop cancer while pregnant and require radiation therapy are generally advised to undergo abortion. The risk to the fetus bombarded by this level of radiation is great indeed.

Diagnostic "Routine" X-Ray Studies

Most common of all, and of greatest concern to you, are the routine X-ray studies that are intrinsic to modern medicine. You may have a problem that requires X-ray evaluation even though you are pregnant. Or you may not know you are pregnant until after you've had a battery of X-ray studies. Finally, you may need an X-ray study that is unique to pregnant women—X-ray pelvimetry—which tells the physician how wide your pelvis is, where the baby is located and whether delivery should proceed smoothly. What about cases like these? What do we know about the effects of routine diagnostic X rays of the unborn child, and what should you do if you've had any X-ray examinations?

The amount of radiation from diagnostic X-ray studies is minute compared with the massive quantities from atomic blasts or cancer therapy. Thus, diagnostic X rays are safer than those other forms, but they bring some hazard to the unborn child.

There is no evidence to date showing that diagnostic X rays can produce either fetal deformities or genetic mutations. Remember, however, that mutations may take a number of generations to become apparent. Thus, we can't be sure that X rays don't have that potential. The clearest known risk of "routine" X-ray exposure is childhood cancer. Exposure to the fetus of X rays, even "routine" X rays does increase the risk of developing various childhood cancers, leukemias in particular.[6-9]

The risk seems to increase in proportion to the number of pictures taken and to the time of the pregnancy. One study found that children who were exposed to radiation during the first trimester had an eight-fold increase in the risk of developing cancer during childhood.[6] This same study, and others as well, found a 1½-fold increased risk in children exposed during the later two thirds of intrauterine life.[6-9]

What does this mean in real numbers? It in no way means that all, or even most of those exposed children will get cancer. It simply means that their chances are greater than if they hadn't been exposed. Here are some numbers: the usual incidence of cancers in children ages birth to 9 years is in the order of 7 per 10,000. Those who were exposed to radiation during the first trimester had an 8-fold increase in risk. In other words, 56 out of every 10,000 of those youngsters developed some form of cancer.

Of those who were exposed later in development, the chances were increased by about 50 percent, over the unexposed group. Instead of 7, 10 of every 10,000 of those children got cancer.

In all of these cases, the X-ray exposure to the fetus was direct. In other words, these were films taken of the woman's pelvis, lower back or lower abdomen. These were not chest X rays, dental films or skull films. The farther the baby is from the X-ray site, the less exposure received, and the less the chances for future injury.

Can we translate this into some concrete recommendations for you? Assume you need a large battery of X-ray tests that involve your low back, low abdomen or pelvis, or that you got these unwittingly during the early part of pregnancy. Most authorities would suggest that you consider having an abortion. This is particularly true if you must have what we call "fluoroscopic" studies such as a lower GI or barium enema examination. This type of exam differs from the usual snapshot type in that the radiologist continually looks inside you as the dense white liquid courses through your intestines. The radiation exposure from this sort of study exceeds the average dose from a single picture or two.

Perhaps the thought of an abortion is out of the question for you. Where do you and your baby stand? If you've had two to four X-ray pictures taken, chances are great that your baby won't be injured. Note the figures we gave you earlier. The cancer risk may be far greater in your child than in the X-ray-free youngster, but the odds are still with you—56 in 10,000 or so. And what if you've had more than three X rays or have undergone a fluoroscopic procedure. To date, no one can tell you exactly how dangerous a barium enema examination or a series of 10 lower abdominal films might be. The risk to your child probably increases in proportion to the number of X rays taken, but concrete numbers aren't available. One reason that abortion is urged is that physicians don't want to use you and your child to find out.

X rays of other parts of the body are relatively safe as long as the beam is concentrated at the right place. It is advisable that you wear a lead protective apron over your lower abdomen just to be sure. Often X-ray technicians won't automatically cover your lower abdomen with this protective shield. Let them know that you are pregnant and that you would like the added protection of such a shield. Then you can get a chest X ray, skull X rays, X rays of your arms or legs, dental X rays, etc., if you really need them, with no serious worries. Your child won't be affected.

X-Ray Pelvimetry

As many as 30 percent of pregnant women have X-ray pelvimetry, to measure dimensions of the pelvic bones. These studies are used most often in the woman who has never given birth before, since the doctor is often less sure that her pelvis is large enough to accommodate the baby's exit. Pelvimetry can be a valuable medical tool. There are times when the baby is simply too large to get through the mother's pelvis, and the doctor must find out so that he can plan a cesarean section. There are times when the baby is in a strange position which must be corrected or circumvented by an operative birth. There are times when labor ceases or doesn't go properly. The doctor needs to find out why, and X-ray pelvimetry is a useful tool.

Like any other medical aid, it has its place, but it can be overused. There is no place for "routine" X-ray pelvimetry. It is a procedure that has attendant risks, albeit minimal, and must be reserved for times of need. If your doctor has a good reason to want to get these X-ray studies—for example, he is concerned that the outlet is too narrow for the baby—by all means, let him order the study. In general, the closer to delivery time, the safer for the baby. The risks: we discussed them earlier. Though there is a small increase, from seven to ten per ten thousand, in the incidence of childhood cancer when fetuses are exposed late in pregnancy, this is a small chance to take to help insure a safe delivery.

Sonography

Sonography is a relatively new medical tool. It uses sound waves rather than light waves to see structures buried deep within our bodies. Sonography has been touted as the *safe* alternative to those destructive X rays. This may or may not be true: it's too early to be certain. Remember, it took 30 years after X rays were discovered before their destructive qualities came to light. Sound waves can be injurious to tissues, and although no clearcut human problems have yet been identified, they shouldn't be overused.

In a recent preliminary communication (not yet published in the scientific literature or absolutely corroborated) some German researchers brought up some worrisome observations. They have some early hints that there may be an increased incidence of sterility in young men whose mothers had undergone sonography during the early part of pregnancy. At this point, all we can say is that we'll have to wait and see whether there's any truth to these concerns.

Sonography is used quite freely in pregnant women. Once again, like X rays, it can be a very useful tool. It tells the doctor exactly where the baby and the placenta are located. It helps identify certain abnormalities of placental growth and location. It is invaluable in improving the safety of amniocentesis (the procedure that withdraws amniotic fluid directly through the mother's abdominal wall to carry out special diagnostic studies). Without sonography, the surgeon doesn't know exactly where to put the amniocentesis needle and he might hit the umbilical cord or parts of the placenta which can prove fatal to the baby.

Thus sonography has its place, but don't accept the claim that it is absolutely and unquestionably safe. We just don't know for sure. Don't get a sonogram unless there is a good reason. Too many women are asking to have them made "just for the fun of it." They want that first picture of their baby to be taken before he's born. That may be fun, but its not worth the risk. It's like wiggling those toes under the X-ray machine.

Summary

1. Like drugs, X rays and sonography should not be used indiscriminately in pregnant women. When they are necessary, they are indispensable; when they are not, the hazard to the baby, however small, doesn't justify the risk.

2. Heavy X-ray exposure in lower abdomen, pelvis or low back, particularly during the first third of pregnancy, may warrant having an abortion. If your personal convictions eliminate abortion as an alternative for you, chances are still with you and your baby. If you've had only a few regular films, he runs a higher risk of developing childhood cancers than do unexposed youngsters, but the odds remain strongly in his favor. If you've had many more than that, no one can tell you where he stands.

3. X-ray pelvimetry and sonography are "routine" obstetrical studies. If they are necessary, they are safe enough to accept them willingly. If they are not essential, they aren't worth any possible risk to your unborn child.

XIX

Chemicals at Home and at Work

We live and work in a sea of chemical products: cosmetics, clothing and hair dyes, gardening aids, paints, insecticides, cleaning solutions and thousands of others surround us. Most are so ingrained in our daily lives that they're second nature; we use them without a moment's hesitation or a passing thought; they are simply part of us and our world. It's really remarkable how little we know about the effects of most of these on the human body. They've crept, one by one, from factories to the marketplace with little testing and few controls.

In the past, hazards of a common household product or an industrial chemical or waste have generally remained a secret until major crises alerted the world. Undoubtedly you recall some of them. Vinyl chloride, a common organic chemical that was used extensively as an aerosol spray propellant was abruptly taken off the market recently. The reason: a number of factory workers developed liver cancer that was rather conclusively linked to this chemical.

Chloroform was banned from the 2,000 or so household products and drugs that contained it when studies showed that it could cause cancers in animals. New waste disposal methods were introduced after hundreds of Japanese youngsters were born with cerebral palsy and other birth defects caused by mercury contamination of fish they ate. In Italy, scores of pregnant women who were exposed to dioxin, an industrial waste that causes birth defects, demanded abortions. And the list goes on.

If we know little about the effects of chemicals around us on our own bodies, we know even less about their effects on the unborn child. The link between a chemical and a birth injury is removed by a generation and is much harder to pin down.

Our hope here is to point out some of the potentially hazardous chemicals that you might encounter at work or at home. Most often we won't be able to tell you, "Yes, this is known to be dangerous to the fetus," because no one has looked into it. The best we'll be able to do is to give you what information there is about a chemical and to reach some educated guesses about potential risks. We apologize for our scanty data—far less than the hard data about medications (and even that has a long way to go before it's complete)—but we present what results the inadequate research has yielded. Scientists simply have not focused on the place of the fetus in this increasingly synthetic world.

Our purpose here is the one we introduced in Chapter 1. We don't want you to worry about things that you can't control or remote risks that are totally unknown. Therefore, we will consider only those chemicals that are easily avoidable and/or probably hazardous. We don't want to make you afraid of your environment, but we do want you to be aware of it. We want you to pause a moment before you pick up that can of insect spray, that paint brush dripping with turpentine, the hair dyes and cosmetics that you use automatically.

Household Chemicals

Aerosol Sprays

Before long the aerosol spray can that conquered the marketplace may be a collector's item. Environmentalists are concerned about possible damage to our upper atmosphere and a number of manufacturers, anticipating future controls, have begun to repackage their products. Hair sprays, underarm deodorant sprays, and furniture polishes may soon be housed in simple mechanical pump cans. Until they are, we recommend that you minimize your use of these aerosol cans while you are pregnant. There's no known risk, but here are the concerns:

In the first place, the fluorocarbon propellants, generally thought to be inert and harmless, may not be. They are closely related chemically to the anesthetic gas halothane. Halothane has been implicated in birth defects. A number of studies of nurse anesthetists and female anesthesiologists who were constantly exposed to this gas during pregnancy, found a higher incidence of various congenital malformations.[1-3]

Secondly, these aerosol sprays make a fine mist and release larger amounts of chemical agents than do the pump-type sprays. We don't even know what all of the chemicals in these various products are, but you can be sure that some of them are taken into your lungs, enter your bloodstream and then the body of your growing fetus. Are the other components (besides the fluorocarbon propellent) harmful? No one knows, but why take the chance? It's easy enough to substitute roll-on deodorants, liquid furniture polishes and pump-type hair sprays.

Insecticides and Weed Killers

Refrain from using insecticides and herbicides. Some of those chemicals are known to be absorbed through your lungs or your skin, and they might injure the growing fetus. Let someone else spray the garden, the patio or the kitchen cabinets, and keep away until the fumes have had plenty of time to dissipate.

Paints

Avoid, if you can, painting rooms, particularly with oil-base paints. Don't breathe in turpentine or paint fumes. These petroleum distillates definitely enter the system of anyone who breathes them in. Even if the concentration is too low to hurt you, they may affect your growing child. There's no hard evidence that these products will injure the unborn child, but then again there's no evidence that they won't. We know that these products can be injurious to adults if the concentration is great enough. You may have experienced some dizziness during a past painting chore, so why take a chance with your unborn child?

Cleaning and Polishing Aids

When you clean and polish, wear gloves. Many strong cleaning products contain chemicals that can be absorbed through your skin. When you use ammonia-containing agents, again, be certain that ventilation is adequate. Ammonia is readily taken up by your body. It is also a natural waste product, so you have some built-in protective mechanisms, but too much is toxic to your system.

You don't know how much of these toxic agents you're taking in when you do your normal cleaning chores, so be safe. Use these products carefully, with good ventilation, far away from your face, and with gloves on your hands.

Oven and Drain Cleaners

Most oven and drain cleaners use strong caustic bases—lye, sodium hydroxide and the like—as their working ingredients. Use them cautiously, more for your own protection than for that of your unborn child. If they get into your mouth, your lungs or onto your skin, they can produce severe burns. They won't hurt your baby (unless you actually swallow massive quantities) because your body is well equipped to neutralize those bases and render them harmless.

Cosmetics and Beauty Aids

Even though you rub these on your skin, massage them into your hair or spray them on the outside of your body they can still enter your internal system.

Many chemicals can be absorbed through your skin, get into your bloodstream and be shuttled into your baby's tissues.

Attempting to define the hazards of common cosmetics is like trying to discuss a book after a brief glance at the cover. You see, the ingredients contained in most cosmetics are closely guarded secrets. In the past the only way to expose the secrets was through a lawsuit: an individual would develop some serious reaction to a cosmetic, and would sue the company. In the courtroom the list of ingredients would, of necessity, be revealed.

A 58-year-old woman recently won $325,000 in a settlement with Mitchum-Thayer, Inc., the manufacturer of a skin cream "Fortified Esoterica." It seems that this cosmetic contains mercury, a highly toxic chemical. The woman developed mercury poisoning which permanently affected her speech, memory, hearing and muscle coordination.[4]

We know that mercury is poisonous to the unborn child.[5,6,7] We mentioned earlier the severe retardation, paralysis and congenital deformities mercury poisoning produced in Japanese children. At this point we don't know whether any unborn children have suffered from their mother's unwitting use of poisonous cosmetics, but the possibility is real and alarming.

Soon some of the mysteries surrounding cosmetics will end. The FDA has ruled the cosmetic manufacturers must label their products to let the public know what's in them. You'll be able to read the labels, just as you do with foods and drugs, and make some intelligent choices. Avoid any cosmetics that contain mercury, arsenic or lead when you are pregnant. They're all toxic to the growing embryo and fetus.[7]

Since the other ingredients are currently a secret, you'll have to check with your doctor about their safety once the detailed labels appear. Assume that they're entering your body, just as if you swallowed them. Ask your doctor to check with the FDA or the Maternal and Child Welfare section of the National Institutes of Health to see what is known about their effects on the growing child.

Avoid all hair dyes during pregnancy. Ample studies in bacteria and various laboratory animals have shown that the common hair dyes are absorbed through the skin and can affect the cell's genes.[8,9] They are prone to produce gene mutations, and they can also cause cancer. The likelihood is that they can disturb growing embryonic cells, make them go awry and lead to birth defects, though this has not yet been proven conclusively.

Recently, a 52-year-old woman developed aplastic anemia—a fatal disease in which the bone marrow stops making blood cells. The cause: a hair dye containing paraphenylenediamine, one of the most common commercial dyes.[9]

If a hair dye could affect an adult this way, can you imagine the potential threat to that minute embryo or fetus? So let your hair stay its natural color—while you're pregnant, anyway. Hair dyes are almost surely a potential danger for your unborn child.

Occupational Hazards

Certain jobs can be dangerous to the health of both you and your unborn child. Recently the federal government has accepted some responsibility to help insure your safety at work. It has established a regulatory body known as OSHA (Occupational Safety and Health Administration), which is charged with the duty of creating and policing health and safety standards at the workplace.

Many environmental scientists and toxicologists have compiled vast collections of work-exposure information. A number of their publications, available in most libraries, can tell you whether your work environment is dangerous.[10-13] Are the fumes that you inhale day after day injurious? Should you take special precautions while you are at work? If you get sick, could chemicals from work be responsible?

Since the list of chemicals such as organic solvents, dyes, lead, arsenic, paints, insecticides and thousands of others, is so vast, we can't possibly catalogue them here. If you work in a place where chemicals of any kind abound, we would suggest that you take a few moments to look them up in the four books listed in the references to this chapter.[10-13] Read the OSHA regulations and recommendations, and if you have questions write to the Occupational Safety Health Administration in Washington, D.C. Its address and telephone number are listed in the reference section.[14]

What about your unborn child? How does your work environment affect him? As is so often the case, we know a great deal about work and your health, but we know relatively little about effects during pregnancy.

Recently the National Institute for Occupational Safety and Health (NIOSH) indicated in a Senate subcommittee hearing that OSHA and NIOSH were embarking on these vital studies. They had identified at least 20 chemicals that produce or were suspected of producing birth defects. They estimated that more than one million women of childbearing age could be working in hazardous environments. The NIOSH director admitted that "chemicals are regulated, but not with this (protection of women of childbearing ages) in mind." He pledged, however, that new efforts to protect the unborn child were moving full steam ahead. We hope so.

For now, assume that any chemicals in your environment that can injure you can injure your unborn child. He is small, growing and even more vulnerable. It's easy to see that levels in the air or on your skin that might be safe for you, may well be too much for his fragile body to tolerate.

Chemicals that cause cancer, mutations or injuries to specific organs (such as liver or kidney), are likely to be dangerous for the unborn child. In a few cases we know of certain work-related environmental hazards that have been shown to produce birth defects. In other cases, we can only guess that they might.

Women Exposed to Benzene, Toluene and Organic Solvents and Dyes

Many of these compounds are known to produce bladder cancers, leukemia, liver cancers and other liver diseases. If you work in a manufacturing plant that makes them, or in an industrial facility that uses them, you need to exercise extreme caution. The more direct contact you have with these agents, the greater your concerns must be. So, if you're actually in the chemical plant, breathing noxious chemical fumes or, if your hands frequently dip into vats of dye or other dangerous chemicals, you're seriously risking your baby's welfare. If you're a secretary, an executive or a receptionist in a well-ventilated office far removed from the plant, your worries are far less.

Those of you who are pregnant, or expect to be soon, and are employed in this potentially dangerous environment should take some positive steps. See your company's safety officer or occupational health director, explain your situation and request a transfer to a safer location. If you don't get a satisfactory reply consult the OSHA department in Washington, D.C. (address in reference.[14])

Women Exposed to Vinyl Chloride

Vinyl chloride is a common component of plastics and was formerly used as an aerosol propellant. Vinyl chloride workers have developed hepatic angiosarcomas, a type of liver cancer. Although OSHA regulations have markedly improved plant safety, you can't take any chances with this dangerous organic chemical. Don't work in a plant that makes or uses vinyl chloride, while you're pregnant. If you work nearby, make sure the air is free from any contamination. Again, ask the plant safety officer or occupational health consultant to help. If not, OSHA will.

Women Exposed to Metals— Arsenic, Mercury, Lead

These and many other inorganic chemicals and their compounds are teratogenic—they produce a wide variety of birth defects. Don't work with these chemicals, if you are or could be pregnant.

Operating Room Personnel

A number of reports have identified hazards to the offspring of nurse anesthetists and female anesthesiologists.[1-3] Miscarriages and birth deformities are higher in the children of these women. The suspected culprit is halothane, an anesthetic gas, which they frequently use. Though they are careful not to let high concentrations of the gas escape into the air, enough evidently does get into their blood to injure the embryo or fetus.

Other operating room personnel, such as scrub nurses and circulating nurses, may or may not be at risk. Certainly, their exposure is less than that of the women in charge of the anesthetics, but we don't know if it's enough to do harm.

It's a wise idea for nurse anesthetists and anesthesiologists to minimize their exposure to anesthetic gases, particularly during the first three months of pregnancy. If possible, do only the cases that use local, regional or intravenous anesthetic agents.

Traffic Policewomen, Parking Lot Attendants, Auto Mechanics, and Toll Booth Workers

There probably aren't too many of you who spend your days at these jobs, but a few of you undoubtedly do. Furthermore, as women increasingly take their rightful place beside men in the working world, more of you will. What are the similarities among these seemingly different occupations and what are the risks?

The similarities: constant exposure to automobile fumes. The risks: the carbon monoxide and lead which spew from automobile exhaust pipes and can be hazardous to the unborn child.

Two things are certain. First, the lead and carbon monoxide concentrations in the air are exceedingly high in places where there are lots of cars. The more cars, and the less well ventilated the area, the higher the concentrations. Thus the indoor garage attendant, the automobile mechanic and the tunnel worker generally have the highest exposure; the traffic policewomen and toll booth workers less because they are outdoors.

Second, both carbon monoxide and lead can harm the fetus. A variety of congenital deformities and a higher incidence of miscarriages have been linked to these toxins.[15-18] What we don't yet know is the most important piece of information for you. Is the exposure that you might get in these jobs sufficient to threaten your unborn child?

This is one of those occupational-hazard questions that OSHA and NIOSH are currently examining, but the answers are not yet available. The best recommendations for you at this point are: 1) Checks with the government agency listed in reference 14 to find out the latest information. 2) If possible, try to transfer to a less dangerous location. For example, if you are a policewoman, see if you can do non-traffic duties during your pregnancy. 3) If you are in a job that bombards you with exhaust fumes and you can't change jobs or transfer, perhaps you can get a leave of absence for the first three months of your pregnancy. That is probably the most vulnerable period for your unborn child.

Summary

Certain chemicals at work and home can affect your unborn child. Often, you can take simple affirmative steps to lessen the risk. Being aware of your environment, thinking before you use chemicals, considering the type of work exposures you have—these are important steps to insure the safety of your growing child.

NOTES
CHAPTER REFERENCES

Chapters 3 and 4

General References

Apgar, V. A., and J. Beck, *Is My Baby All Right?*, Simon and Schuster Inc., New York (1972).

Barnes, A. C., *Intra-Uterine Development*, Lea and Febiger, Phila. (1968).

Giroud, Antoine, *The Nutrition of the Embryo*, Charles C Thomas, Phila. (1970).

Goss, C. M., ed., *Anatomy of the Human Body* (*Henry Gray*), Lea and Febiger, Phila. (1963).

Hellman, L. M., and J. A. Pritchard, *Williams Obstetrics*, Appleton-Century-Crofts, New York (1971).

Patten, B. M., *Human Embryology*, McGraw Hill, New York (1968).

Williams, P. L., and C. P. Wendell-Smith, *Basic Human Embryology*, J. B. Lippincott Co., Phila., Montreal (1966).

Chapter 5

References Cited

1. Simpson, J. W., R. W. Lawless, and A. C. Mitchell, *Obstetrics and Gynecology*, 45: 481 (1975).

2. Winick, M., ed., *Nutrition and Fetal Development*, John Wiley and Sons, New York (1974).

3. Lechtig, A., H. Delgado, R. E. Lasky, R. E. Klein, P. L. Engle, C. Yarborough, and J. P Habicht, *Am. J. Dis. Child.* 129: 434 (1975).

4. Naeye, R. L., W. Blanc, and C. Paul, *Pediatrics* 52: 494 (1973).

5. Stein, Z., and M. Susser, *Pediatr. Res.* 9: 76 (1975).

6. Jacobson, H. N., *Clinical Perinatology* (1975).

7. Iyenger, L., *Am. J. Obst. and Gynecol.* 102: 834 (1968).

8. Ravelli, G. P., Z. A. Stein, and M. W. Susser, *New Eng. J. Med.* 295: 349 (1976).

9. Adams, M. S., and J. D. Niswander, *Human Biol.* 40: 226 (1968).

10. Churchill, J. A., *Current Research in Chronic Neurologic Dis. of Children. Merrill Palmer Quart. Behav. Develop.* 9: 95 (1963).

11. Churchill, J. A., M. A. Neff, and D. F. Caldwell, *Obstetrics and Gynecology* 28: 425 (1966).

12. Caldwell, D. F., and Churchill, J. A. *Neurology* 17: 95 (1967).

13. Leitch, I., *Proc. Nutr. Soc.* (*London*) 16: 38 (1957).

14. Burke, B. S., V. A., S. B. Kirkwood, and H. C. Stuart, *Amer. J. Obstetr. and Gynecol.* 46: 38 (1943).

15. Ebbs, J. H., F. F. Tisdall, and W. A. Scott, *J. Nutrition* 22: 515 (1941).

16. Dieckmann, W. J., D. F. Turner, E. J. Meiller, L. J. Savage, A. J. Hill, M. F. Straube, R. E. Pottinger, and L. M. Rynkiewicz, *J. Amer. Diet. Assn.* 27: 1046 (1951).

17. Berry, K. and D. G. Wiehl, *Milbank Mem. Fund. Quart.* 30: 119 (1952).

18. Jeans, P. C., M. B. Smith, and G. Stearns, *J. Amer. Diet. Assn.* 31: 576 (1955).

19. Woodhill, M. M., A. S. van den Berg, B. S. Burke, and F. J. Stare, *Amer. J. Obstet. and Gynecol.* 70: 987 (1955).

20. Kasius, R. U., A. Randall, W. T. Tompkins, and D. G. Wiehl, *Milbank Mem. Fund. Quart.* 36: 335 (1958).

21. Butler, N., in *Nutrition and Fetal Development:* 173, M. Winick ed., John Wiley and Sons, New York (1974).

22. Babson, S. G., and J. Kangas, N. Young, and J. L. Bramhall, *Pediatrics* 45: 937 (1970).

23. Chase, H. C., *National Center for Health Statistics,* Series 3, No. 6, US Dept. HEW, Washington, D.C.

24. Stein, Z., M. Susser, G. Saenger, and F. Marolla, *Science* 178: 708 (1972).

25. Livingston, R. B., Report to the Fifth Annual Meeting of Society of Neurosciences based on Ten State Nutritional Survey by Center for Disease Control (1976).

26. Brasel, J. A., R. A. Ehrenkranz, and M. Winick, *Devel. Biol.* 23: 424 (1970).

27. Fish, I., and M. Winick, *Exp. Neurol.* 25: 534 (1969).

28. Winick, M., *Am. J. Obst. and Gynecol.* 109: 166 (1971).

29. Dobbing, J., *Am. J. Dis. Child.* 120: 411 (1970).

30. Bergner, L. and M. W. Susser, *Pediatrics* 46: 944 (1970).

31. Rush, D., and P. Fergus, *Abstr. Am. Pediatr. Soc.* April (1969).

32. Rush, D. in *The Problem of Congenital Defects, New Directions,* D. T. Janerich, R. G. Skalko, and I. H. Porter, eds. Academic Press, New York (1973).

33. Davie, R., N. Butler and H. Goldstein, *From Birth to Seven.* Longmans, London (1972).

34. *Maternal Nutrition and The Course of Pregnancy,* Committee on Maternal Nutrition Food and Nutrition Board National Research Council, National Academy of Sciences, Washington, D.C. (1970).

35. Aznar, R., and A. E. Bennett, *Amer. J. Obstet. and Gynecol.,* 81: 934 (1961).

36. Hassan, A. M., and F. H. Falls, *Amer. J. Obstet. and Gynecol.,* 88: 256 (1964).

37. King, J. C., D. H. Calloway, and S. Margen, *J. Nutr.* 103: 772 (1973).
38. McCance, R. A., and E. M. Widdowson, *Proc. Royal Soc. London* 185: 1 (1974).

General References

Catz, C. S., *Nutrition as an Environmental Factor from the Pediatric Viewpoint* in International Conference on Environmental Health, Primosten, Yugoslavia (Oct. 1973).

Committee on Maternal Nutrition: Maternal Nutrition and the Course of Pregnancy, Washington, D.C., National Academy of Sciences (1970).

McCance, R. A., and E. M. Widdowson, *The Determinants of Growth and Form* in *Proc. Royal Soc. London* 185: 1 (1974).

Pitkin, R. M., *Obstetrics and Gynecology* in *Nutritional Support of Medical Practice,* C. E. Anderson, D. B. Coursin, and H. A. Schneider, eds., Harper and Row, Hagerstown, Md. (1975).

Pitkin, R. M., *Risks Related to Nutritional Problems in Pregnancy,* in *Risks in the Practice of Modern Obstetrics,* S. Aladjem, ed., C. V. Mosby, Saint Louis (1975).

Pitkin, R. M., H. A. Kaminetsky, M. Newton and J. A. Pritchard, *Maternal Nutrition: A Selective Review of Clinical Topics,* in *Obstet. Gynecol.* 40: 773 (1972).

Nutrition and Fetal Development, M. Winick, ed. John Wiley and Sons, New York (1974).

Nutrition in Pregnancy and Lactation, Report of a WHO expert Committee, WHO Tech. Rep. Ser. 302: 1-54 (1965).

Thomson, A. M., and F. E. Hytten, *Nutrition During Pregnancy* in *Food Nutrition and Health. World Review of Nutrition and Dietetics,* 16: 22 (1973).

Chapter 6

References Cited

1. Horowitz, I., E. M. Fabry, and C. D. Gerson, *J. Amer. Med. Assn.* 235; 2624 (1976).
2. Heller, S., R. M. Salkeld, and W. F. Korner, *Amer. J. Clin. Nutr.* 26: 1339 (1973).
3. Pitkin, R. M. in *Risks in the Practice of Modern Obstetrics,* S. Aladjem, ed.: 165, C. V. Mosby Co., Saint Louis (1975).
4. Friedman, W. R., and C. M. Roberts, *Circulation* 34:77 (1966).
5. Taussig, H. B., *Ann. Intern. Med.* 65: 1195 (1966).

General References

Committee on Maternal Nutrition: Maternal Nutrition and the Course of Pregnancy, Washington, D.C., National Academy of Sciences (1970).

Pitkin, R. M., Obstetrics and Gynecology, in *Nutritional Support of Medical Practice,* C. E. Anderson, D. B. Coursin, and H. A. Schneider, eds., Harper and Row, Hagerstown, Md. (1975).

The Pharmacological Basis of Therapeutics, L. S. Goodman and A. Gilman, eds., fourteenth ed., The Macmillan Co., New York (1975).

Pitkin, R. M., *Risks Related to Nutritional Problems* in *Risks in the Practice of Modern Obstetrics,* S. Aladjem, ed., C. V. Mosby Co., Saint Louis (1975).

Pitkin, R. M., Vitamins and Minerals in Pregnancy, *Clin. Perinatol.* 2: 221 (1975).

Pitkin, R. M., H. A. Kaminetzky, H. A. Newton, and J. A. Pritchard, Maternal Nutrition: a selective review of Clinical Topics, *Obstet. Gynecol.* 40: 773 (1972).

Nutrition and Fetal Development, M. Winick, ed., John Wiley and Sons, New York (1974).

Reference Guides

Bowes, A. de P., and C. F. Church, *Food Values of Portions Commonly Used,* eleventh ed., J. P. Lippincott, Philadelphia, Toronto (1970).

Food and Nutrition Board: Recommended Dietary Allowances, ed. 8, Washington, D.C., National Academy of Sciences (1974).

Guthrie, H. A., *Introductory Nutrition,* second ed., C. V. Mosby Co., Saint Louis (1971).

Chapter 7

General References

Adamsons, K., and I. Joelsson, The Effects of Pharmacological Agents Upon the Fetus and Newborn, *Am. J. Obstet. and Gynecol.* 96: 437 (1966).

Apgar, V., and J. Beck, *Is My Baby All Right?* Simon and Schuster Co., New York (1972).

Barnes, A. C., The Fetal Environment: Drugs and Chemicals, ch. 19 in *Intra Uterine Development,* A. C. Barnes, ed., Lea and Febiger, Philadelphia, Pa. (1968).

Catz, C. S., and D. Abuelo, Drugs and Pregnancy, *Drug Therapy,* p. 79 (April 1974).

Fetal Pharmacology, L. O. Boreus, ed., Raven Press, New York (1973).

Goldstein, A., L. Aronow, and S. M. Kalman, *Principles of Drug Action,* Harper and Row, New York (1974).

Nishimura, H., and T. Tanimura, *Clinical Aspects of the Teratogenicity of Drugs,* American Elsevier Co., New York (1976).

The Pharmacological Basis of Therapeutics, L. S. Goodman and A. Gilman, eds., fourteenth ed., The Macmillan Co., New York (1975).

Physicians' Desk Reference, Medical Economics Co., Oradell, N.J. (1976).

Rosen, M. G. and L. Rosen, *In the Beginning: Your*

Baby's Brain Before Birth, A Plume Book, New American Library, New York (1975).

Yaffe, S. J., and C. S. Catz, Drugs and the Intrauterine Patient, ch. 6: 125 in *Risks in the Practice of Modern Obstetrics,* S. Aladjem, ed., C. V. Mosby Co., Saint Louis (1975).

Chapter 8

References Cited

1. Hill, R. M., *Clin. Pharmacol. Ther.,* 14: 654 (1973).
2. Medalie, J. H., D. Serr, H. N. Neufeld, M. Brown, N. Berandt, M. Sternberg, P. Sive, S. Schoenfeld, Z. Fuchs, and S. Karo, *Adv. Exp. Med. Biol.* 27: 481 (1972).
3. Nelson, M. M., and J. O. Forfar, *Br. Med. J.* 1: 52 (1971).
4. Wegman, M., *Pediatrics,* 56: 960 (1975).
5. Degenhardt, K. H., H. Kerken, K. Knorr, S. Koller, and H. R. Wiedemann, *Adv. Exp. Med. Biol.* 27: 467 (1972).
6. Villumsen, A. L., *Ugeskr. Laeger* 132: 2179 (1970).
7. Editorial comment, Pediatrics 51: 29 (1973).
8. Medical News, *J. Amer. Med. Ass.* 234: 264 (1975)
9. Wilson, J. G., Acta Endocr. Suppl. 166: 261 (1972).
10. Lenz, W., *Deutsche Med. Wochenschr.* 86: 2555 (1961).
11. Williams, R. T., *Lancet* 1: 723 (1963).
12. McBride, W. G., *Med. J. Autral.* 2: 689 (1963).
13. Lenz, W., *Ann. N.Y. Acad. Sci.* 123: 228 (1965).
14. Stolley, P. D., *Internat. J. Health Services* 4: 131 (1974).
15. Vaux, N. W., and A. D. Rakoff, *Am J. Obstet. Gynecol.* 50: 354 (1945).
16. Smith, O. W., *Am. J. Obstet. Gynecol.* 56: 821 (1948).

17. Herbst, A. L., H. Ulfelder, and D. C. Poskanzer, *N. Eng. J. Med.* 284: 878 (1971).

18. Noller, K. L., D. G. Decker, M. B. Dockerty, A. P. Lanier, R. A. Smith and R. E. Simmonds, *Obstetr. and Gynecol.* 43: 640 (1974).

19. Greenwald, P., P. C. Nasca, W. S. Burnett and A. Polan, *Cancer* 31: 568 (1973).

20. Forsberg, J. G., *Am. J. Obstet. Gynecol.* 113: 83 (1972).

21. Stafl, A., R. F. Mattingly, D. V. Foley and W. C. Fetherston, *Obstetr. and Gynecol.* 43: 118 (1974).

22. Scott, J. W., D. Seckinger and W. Puente-Duany, *J. Reprod. Med.* 12: 187 (1974).

23. Herbst, A. L., R. E. Scully, S. J. Robboy and D. C. Poskanzer, *Progress in Gynecol.* 4: 647 (1975).

24. Herbst, A. L., S. J. Robboy, R. E. Scully and D. C. Poskanzer, *Amer. J. Obstet. Gynecol.* 119: 713 (1974).

General References

See References for Chapter 7

Chapter 9

References Cited

1. McNiel, J. R., *Clin. Pediat.* 12: 347 (1973).

2. Carter, M. P. and F. Wilson, *Lancet* 1: 1267 (1963).

3. Richards, I. D. G., *Brit. J. Prevent. Soc. Med.* 23: 218 (1969).

4. Nelson, M. M., and J. O. Forfar, *Brit. Med. J.* 1: 523 (1971).

5. Klemetti, A., and L. Saxen, *The Finnish Register of Congenital Malformations Health Services Research of the National Board of Health in Finland,* Helsinki (1970).

6. Bleyer, W. A., and R. T. Breckenridge, *J. Amer. Med. Assn.* 213: 2049 (1970).

7. Corby, D. G., and I. Schulman, *J. Pediatr.* 79: 307 (1971).

8. Corby, D. G., C. L. Zirbel, M.S. Gibson and I. Schulman, *Clin. Toxicol.* 6: 300 (1973).

9. Collins, E., and G. Turner, *Lancet* 2: 335 (1975).

10. Turner, G., and E. Collins, *Lancet* 2: 338 (1975).

11. Warnaky, J. and E. Tahacs, *Amer. J. Path.* 35: 315 (1959).

12. Erikksson, M., *Acta Path. Microbiol. Scand.* 76: 164 (1969).

13. Trasler, D. G., *Lancet* 1: 606 (1965).

14. Wilson, J. G., *Fed. Proc.* 30: 104 (1971).

15. Nishimura, H., and T. Tanimura, *Clinical Aspects of the Teratogenicity of Drugs,* pp. 204–209, American Elsevier Pub. Co., New York (1976).

16. Kimmel, C. A., J. G. Wilson, and H. J. Schumacher, *Teratology* 4: 15 (1971).

17. Bovet-Nitti, F., G. Bignami and D. Bovet, *Life Sci.* 5: 303 (1963).

18. Goldstein A., and M. M. Hazel, *Endocrinol.* 56: 215 (1955).

19. King, C. T. G., S. A. Weaver and J. E. Derr, *Amer. J. Obstet. Gynecol.* 93: 563 (1965).

20. King, C. T. G., S. A. Weaver and S. A. Narrod, *J. Pharmacol. Expt. Therap.* 147: 391 (1965).

21. Courtney, K. D. and D. A. Valerio, *Teratology* 1: 163 (1968).

22. Posner, H. S., *Food Cosmet. Toxicol.* 10: 839 (1972).

23. Naranjo, P., and E. Naranjo, *Arzneimitt.-Forsch* 18: 188 (1968).

24. Watson, H., *Brit. Med. J.* 2: 1610 (1962).

25. Pettersson, F., *Lancet* 1: 675 (1964).

26. Smithells, R. W., and E. R. Chinn, *Brit. Med. J.* 1: 217 (1964).

27. Mellin, G. W., and M. Katzenstein, *Lancet* 1: 222 (1963).

28. Yerushalmy, J., and L. Milkovich, *Amer. J. Obstet. Gynecol.* 93: 553 (1965).

Chapter 11

References Cited

1. Desmond, M. M., A. Rudolph, R. M. Hill, J. L. Claghorn, P. R. Dreesen, and I. Burgdorff, Symposium on Mental Retardation, Texas Institute of Medical Sciences, Austin, Texas: University of Texas Press (1969).

2. Butler, N. R., H. Goldstein and E. M. Ross, *Brit. Journ. of Med.* 4: 573 (1972).

3. Meyer, M. B., and G. W. Comstock, *Amer. Journ. Epidemiol.* 96: 1 (1972).

4. Yerushalmy, J., *Amer. J. Obstet. Gynecol.* 112: 277 (1972).

5. Rush, D., and E. H. Kass, *Amer. J. Epidemiol.* 96: 183 (1972).

6. Stevenson, R. E., *The Fetus and the Newborn Infant,* C. V. Mosby Co., Saint Louis (1973).

7. Russell, C. S., R. Taylor, and C. E. Law, *Br. J. Prev. Soc. Med.* 22: 119 (1968).

8. Andrews, J., and J. M. McGarry, *Obstet. Gynaecol. Br. Commonw.* 79: 1057 (1972).

9. Lubs, M. E., *Am. J. Obstet. Gynecol.* 115: 66 (1973).

10. Yerushalmy, J., *Am. J. Epidemiol.* 93: 443 (1971).

11. Lowe, C. R., *Brit. Med. J.* 2: 673 (1959).

12. Fredrick, J., E. D. Alberman, and H. Goldstein, *Nature* 231: 529 (1971).

13. Hook, E. B., *Teratology* 7: A17 (1973).

14. Jones, K. L., D. W. Smith, C. N. Ulleland, and A. P. Streissguth, *Lancet* 1: 1267 (1973).

15. Palmer, R. H., E. M. Ouelette, L. Warner, and S. R. Leichtman, *Pediatrics* 53: 490 (1974).

16. Jones, K. L., D. W. Smith, A. P. Streissguth, and N. C. Myrianthopoulos, *Lancet* 1: 1076 (1974).

17. Green, H. G., *Am. J. Obstet. Gynecol.* 118: 713 (1974).

18. Nishimura, H., and K. Nakai, *Proc. Soc. Exp. Biol. Med.* 104: 140 (1960).

19. Mulvihill, J. J., *Teratology* 8: 69 (1973).

20. Gilbert, E. F., and W. R. Pistey, *J. Reprod. Fertil.* 34: 495 (1973).
21. Health Research Group Survey of Tranquilizer Use in Pregnancy, Washington, D.C. (1976).
22. Milkovich, L., and B. J. van den Berg, *N. Eng. J. Med.* 291: 1268 (1974).
23. Saxen, I., *Int. J. Epidemiol.* 4: 37 (1975).
24. Safra, M. J., and G. P. Oakley, *Lancet* 2: 478 (1975).
25. Hartz, S. C., O. P. Heinomen, and S. Shapiro, et al, *N. Eng. J. Med.* 292: 726 (1975).
26. FDA Drug Bulletin, September-November 1975, Washington, D.C.
27. Rosanelli, K., *Geburtshilfe Frauenheilkd* 30: 713 (1970).
28. Idanpaan-Heikkila, J. E., E. I. Jouppila, J. O. Puolakka and M.S. Vorne, *Am. J. Obstet. Gynecol.* 109: 1011 (1971).
29. Bitnum, S., *Can. Med. Assn. J.* 100: 351 (1969).
30. Zelson, C., E. Rubio, and E. Wasserman, *Pediatrics* 48: 178 (1971).
31. Naeya, R. L., W. Blanc, W. Leblanc, and M. A. Khatamee, *J. Pediatr.* 83: 1055 (1973).
32. Kandall, S. R., *Drug Therapy,* p. 47 (May 1976).
33. Kasirsky, G., and M. F. Tansy, *Teratology* 4: 131 (1971).
34. Nora, J. J., D. G. Trasler, and F. C. Fraser, *Lancet* 2: 1021 (1965).
35. Nora, J. J., A. H. Nora, R. J. Sommerville, R. M. Hill, and D. G. McNamara, *J. Am. Med. Assn.* 202: 1065 (1967).
36. Nora, J. J., T. A. Vargo, A. H. Nora, K. E. Love, and D. G. McNamara, *Lancet* 1: 1290 (1970).
37. Levin, J. N., *J. Pediatr.* 79: 130 (1971).
38. Pace, H. B., W. M., Davis, and L. A. Borgen eds., *Teratogenesis and Marijuana, Ann. N. Y. Acad. Sci.,* 191 (1971).
39. Borgen, L. A., W. M. Davis, and H. B. Pace, *Toxicol. appl. Pharmacol.* 20: 480 (1971).
40. Haley, S. L., P. L. Wright, J. B. Plank, M. L.

Keplinger, M. C. Braude, and J. C. Calandre, *Toxicol. Appl. Pharmacol.* 25: 450 (1973).

41. Alexander, G. J., G. M. Gold, B. E. Miles, and R. B. Alexander, *J. Pharmacol. Exp. Ther.* 173: 48 (1970).

42. Auerbach, R., and J. A. Rugowski, *Science* 157: 1325 (1967).

43. Jacobson, C. B., and C. M. Berlin, *J. Am. Med. Assn.* 222: 1367 (1972).

44. Berlin, C. M., and C. B. Jacobson, *Pediatr. Res.* 4: 377 (1970).

Chapter 12

References Cited

1. Robinson, G. C., and K. G. Cambon, *New Eng. J. Med.* 271: 949 (1964).

2. Kline, A. H., R. J. Blattner, and M. Lunin, *J. Am. Med. Assn.* 188: 178 (1964).

3. Sutherland, J. M., *Amer. J. Dis. Child.* 97: 761 (1959).

4. Dunn, P. M., *J. Obstet. Gynaecol. Brit. Commonw.*, 71: 128 (1964).

5. Perkins, R. P., *Am. J. Obstet. Gynecol.* 111: 379 (1971).

6. Palomaki, J. C., and R. M. Zollinger, Risks in the Management of Surgical Complications of Pregnancy ch. 7: 159 in *Risks in the Practice of Modern Obstetrics*, S. Aladjem ed., C. V. Mosby Co., St. Louis (1975).

7. Rodriguez, S. U., S. L. Leikin, and M. C. Hiller, *New Eng. J. Med.* 270: 881 (1964).

8. Dahl, M., and M. Sillanapaa, Duodecim 81: 309 (1965).

9. Warrell, D. W., and R. Taylor, *Lancet* 1: 117 (1968).

10. Guilbeau, J. A., *Am. J. Obstet. Gynecol.* 65: 227 (1953).

11. Schatz, M., R. Patterson, Z. Stanley, J. O'Rourke,

and H. Melam, *J. Amer. Med. Assn.* 233: 804 (1975).

12. Zellweger, H., *Clin. Pediatr.* 13: 338 (1974).

13. Spiedel, B. D., and S. R. Meadow, *Lancet* 2: 839 (1972).

14. Lowe, C. R., *Lancet* 1: 9 (1973).

15. Fredrick, J., *Brit. Med. J.* 2: 442 (1973).

16. Hirsh, J., J. F. Cade, and A. S. Gallus, *Am. Heart J.* 83: 301 (1972).

17. Tejani, N., *Obstet and Gynecol.* 42: 785 (1973).

18. Hellman, L. M., and J. A. Pritchard, *Williams Obstetrics,* fourteenth ed., Appleton-Century-Crofts, New York (1971).

Chapter 13

References Cited

1. Haire, D., *The Cultural Warping of Childbirth,* International Childbirth Education Association, Hillside, New Jersey 07205 (1972).

2. Hellman, L. M., and J. A. Pritchard, *Williams Obstetrics,* fourteenth ed., Appleton-Century-Crofts, New York (1971).

3. Yaffe, S. J., and C. S. Katz, *Drugs in the Intrauterine Patient* ch. 6: 125 in *Risks in the Practice of Modern Obstetrics,* S. Aladjem ed., C. V. Mosby Co,. St. Louis (1975).

4. Wegman, M., *Pediatrics* 56: 960 (1975).

5. Bowes, W., et al, *Monographs of the Society for Research in Child Development,* 35: 137 (1970).

6. Brazelton, T. B., *J. Pediatr.,* 58: 513 (1961).

7. Khron, R., *Pediatrics* 37: 1012 (1966).

8. Lewis, M., et al, *Amer. J. Dis. Child.* 113: 461 (1967).

9. Ostapowicz, F., *Anesthesia and Analgesia During Labor and Delivery,* Amer. College of Obstetricians and Gynecologists, Chicago, Ill.

10. Lurie, A. D., and J. B. Weiss, *Am. J. Obstetr. Gynecol.* 106: 850 (1970).

11. Asling, J. H., S. M. Shnider, A. J. Margolis, G. L. Wilkinson, and E. L. Way, *Am. J. Obstetr. Gynecol.* 107: 626 (1970).
12. Burt, R. A. P., *Br. J. Anaesth.* 43: 824 (1971).
13. Rogers, R. E., *Am. J. Obstetr. Gynecol.* 106: 913 (1970).

Chapter 14

References Cited

1. Weller, T. J., C. A. Alford, and F. A. Neva, *Yale J. Biol. Med.* 37: 455 (1965).
2. Forbes, J. A., *Am. J. Dis. Child.* 118: 5 (1969).
3. Hellman, L. A., and J. A. Pritchard, *Williams Obstetrics,* fourteenth ed., Appleton-Century-Crofts, New York (1971).
4. Greenhill, J. P., and E. A. Freedman, *Biological Principles and Modern Practice of Obstetrics,* W. B. Saunders and Co., Philadelphia (1974).
5. Cooper, L. Z., *Rubella: a preventable cause of birth defects,* in *Intrauterine infections* D. Bergsma ed., Original Articles Series, 4: 7, pp. 23-25, National Foundation (1968).
6. Plotz, E. J., *N. Y. State J. Med.* 65: 1239 (1965).
7. Rambar, A. C., *Ill. Med. J.* 136: 599 (1969).
8. Brown, A. K., and J. G. Freehafer, *Prenatal Risks: a pediatrician's point of view,* in *Risks in the Practice of Modern Obstetrics,* S. Aladjem ed., C. V. Mosby Co., St. Louis (1975).
9. Editorial comment, *The Lancet* p. 769, (October 6, 1973).
10. Meyer, H. M., and P. D. Parkman, *J. Am. Med. Assn.* 215: 613 (1971).
11. Harris, J. W., *J. Am. Med. Assn.* 72: 978 (1919).
12. Moloshok, R. E., *Clin. Obstet. Gynecol.* 9: 608 (1966).
13. Christensen, P. E., et al, *Acta Med. Scand.* 144: 431 (1953).
14. Siegler, M. A., and H. Keyser, *Am. J. Obstet. Gynecol.* 86: 1068 (1963).

15. Overall J. C., and L. A. Glasgow, *J. Pediatr.* 77: 315 (1970).

Chapter 16

References Cited

1. Desmonts, G., J. Couvreur, and B. Rachid, *Arch. Fr. Proc.* 22: 1183 (1969).
2. Nelson, W., V. Vaughn and R. J. McKay eds., *Textbook of Pediatrics*, edition 9, W. B. Saunders and Co., Philadelphia (1969).
3. Frenkel, J. K., *BioScience* 23: 343 (1973).
4. Couvreur, J., in *Hentsch, Toxoplasmosis* 119, Hans Huber, Bern (1971).
5. Desmonts, G., and J. Couvreur, *Rapports* 3: 453 (1967).

Chapter 17

General References

How Safe is Safe? The Design of Policy on Drugs and Food Additives, First Academy Forum, National Academy of Sciences, Washington, D.C. (1974).

Ingelfinger, F. J., *New Eng. J. Med.* 293: 1319 (1975).

Nishimura, H., and T. Tanimura, *Clinical Aspects of the Teratogenicity of Drugs*, American Elsevier Publishing Co., New York (1976).

Sweeteners: Issues and Uncertainties, Fourth Academy Forum, National Academy of Sciences, Washington, D.C. (1975).

Toxicants Occurring Naturally in Foods, Committee on Food Protection, Food and Nutrition Board National Research Council, National Academy of Sciences, Washington, D.C. (1973).

The Use of Chemicals in Food Production, Processing, Storage and Distribution, Committee on Food Protection, Food and Nutrition Board Division of Biology and Agriculture National Research Council, National Academy of Sciences, Washington, D.C. (1973).

Whelan, E., and F. Stare, *Panic in the Pantry*, Atheneum Press, New York (1975).

Chapter 18

References Cited

1. Barnes, A. C., ed., Irradiation, ch. 20, in *Intra Uterine Development,* Lea and Febiger, Philadelphia, Pa. (1968).
2. Miller, R. W., *Pediatrics* 18: 1 (1956).
3. Plummer, G. W., *Pediatrics* 10: 687 (1952).
4. Neel, J. V., and W. J. Schull, *Science* 128: 343 (1958).
5. Le Vann, L. J., *Alberta Med. Bull.* (1965).
6. Stewart, A., and G. W. Kneale, *The Lancet* 1: 1185 (1970).
7. MacMahon, B., *J. Natl. Canc. Inst.* 28: 1173 (1962).
8. Stewart, A., et al., *The Lancet* 2: 447 (1956).
9. Townsend, L., *Med. J. Australia* 2: 289 (1958).

Chapter 19

References Cited

1. Cohen, E. N., J. W. Bellville, and B. W. Brown, *Anesthesiology* 35: 343 (1971).
2. Ad Hoc Committee on the Effect of Trace Anesthetics on the Health of Operating Room Personnel, American Society of Anesthesiologists, E. N. Cohen, chairman (1974).
3. Corbett, T. H., R. G. Cornell, J. L. Endres, and K. Lieding, *Anesthesiology* 41: 341 (1974).
4. *Hertnagel v. Mitchum-Thayer, Inc.*, Wash., King Cty. Super. Ct. No. 777438, Jan. 1976, ATLA News Letter 19: 69 (Mar. 1976).

5. Vostal, J. J., and T. W. Clarkson, *J. Occup. Med.* 15: 649 (1973).

6. Matsumoto, H., G. Koya, and T. Takeuchi, *J. Neuropath. exp. Neurol.* 24: 563 (1965).

7. Nishimura, H., and T. Tanimura, *Clinical Aspects of The Teratogenicity of Drugs,* American Elsevier Publishing Co., New York (1976).

8. Toghill, P. J., and R. G. Wilcox, *Brit. Med. J.* 1: 502 (1976).

9. Clin-Alert, No. 71, April 16, 1976.

10. *Toxic and Hazardous Industrial Chemicals Safety Manual for Handling and Disposal with Toxicity and Hazard Data,* International Technical Information Institute, Japan (1975).

11. Stellman, J. M., and S. M. Daum, *Work is Dangerous to your Health: a Handbook of Health Hazards in the Workplace and What You Can Do About Them,* Pantheon Books, New York (1973).

12. Sax, I. N., *Dangerous Properties of Industrial Materials,* Litton Educational Publishing, New York (1975).

13. U.S. Department of HEW, *Occupational Diseases: A Guide to their Recognition,* W. M. Gafafer, ed., PHS Pub. no. 1097, Washington, D.C., Government Printing Office (1966).

14. Occupational Safety Health Administration, Department of Labor, Information Services, 200 Constitution Avenue, NW, Washington, D.C. Tel. (202) 523-8148.

15. Muller, G. L., and S. Graham, *New Eng. J. Med.* 252: 1075 (1955).

16. Curtis, G. W., E. J. Algeri, A. J. McBay, and R. Ford, *Arch. Path.* 59: 677 (1955).

17. Goyer, R. A., and B. C. Rhyne, *Int. Rev. expt. Path.* 12: 1 (1973).

18. Palmisano, P. A., R. C. Sneed, and G. Cassady, *J. Pediatr.* 75: 869 (1969).

APPENDIX

Known or Suspected Risks of Various Drugs Taken During Pregnancy

In this section we list a large number of drugs that you might confront during your pregnancy. Some are sold over-the-counter without a doctor's prescription. Some require authorization from your physician. The list includes some brand names (capitalized). These are the actual trade names that the company has given to its drug. It also includes many generic or chemical names. Some of these chemicals may be found in many brand-name drugs, others are unique to a single brand. For example: diazepam is sold as Valium. This is the only brand of the drug diazepam. Aspirin, on the other hand, is found in literally hundreds of different brand-name drugs—Anacin, Bufferin, Excedrin, Coricidin, Sine-Aid, Vanquish and many more.

The following table may seem confusing or even alarming at first glance. Because it is complex and needs to be properly understood to be useful to you, we will spend a few moments here explaining its purpose, meaning and interpretation.

We have divided pregnancy into four segments: the first trimester; the second trimester; the third trimester, and labor and delivery. We have done this for reasons that were discussed throughout the book—the unborn child has unique sensitivities to drugs at different periods along the way.

The notations—?, +, ++, +++, ++++—represent what we know about these drugs. Many of them have been discussed earlier in the text, and you should refer to the relevant chapters for more detailed information.

? means that the drug has been studied very little regarding its effects on the unborn child, and we don't know enough to give specific advice.

+ means that some studies have been performed and thus far the drug has not been shown to be dangerous.

++ means that the drug has been studied and may be dangerous, or that theoretical considerations about the drug make risks a real possibility.

+++ means that the drug or related drugs are probably risky. In some cases this assessment is based on hard laboratory data; in others it is supported by strong theoretical likelihood.

++++ means that the drug is known to present certain risks to the unborn child. Generally these risks have been well-defined, and most are discussed in earlier chapters.

Let us clarify a few points about these classifications and warnings. In the first place, the risk-benefit concept that we have discussed many times must always be applied. Thus, if you urgently need a drug that has ++++ you have got to take it, but only with the guidance and recommendation of your physician. Secondly, all drugs with the same number of plus signs are not equally dangerous. The plus signs tell you how certain we are about the risks, but they do not tell you how great the risks are or what the probability is that these drugs will hurt your child. Thus, we know that aspirin can cause serious problems, particularly near delivery, but the chances that it will do so are not enormous. Chloramphenicol, on the other hand, will cause serious problems in a higher frequency of cases. Both aspirin and chloramphenicol are denoted in column four with ++++.

Finally, the risk will vary depending upon the dosage. Certain vitamins are given +++. This only applies to excessive dosages that greatly exceed those recommended in Chapter 6. The narcotics, barbiturates, amphetamines and other abused drugs vary greatly in risk, depending upon dosage. "Small" refers to occasional therapeutic dosages. "Large" refers to addictive chronic usage.

Monitoring is also important. Note, for example, that the narcotics (morphine, Demerol, codeine, pentazocine) and the anesthetics like halothane and cyclopropane get bad marks—+++ or ++++—during labor and delivery. That is because, as we discussed in chapter 13, they all depress the baby and can lead to serious problems. However, that doesn't mean they can never be used. In chapter 13 we told you that these drugs could be used with relative safety if they were given in controlled dosages and monitored very carefully by skilled obstetricians or anesthesiologists.

In general, the plus signs become more meaningful the longer you take the drug and the greater the dosage. Thus, Valium, aspirin and those others that are noted +++ or ++++ are far less dangerous if you take them a few times than if you take them for months at a time.

Many of the drugs on this list are combination drugs —they contain a number of ingredients. We've marked them according to their most worrisome ingredient. The +++ and ++++ of many of the over-the-counter sleeping, pain, sinus and cold remedies were awarded because of the aspirin they contain.

Before you take any drug, check with your doctor. Ask him or look on the bottle (in those over-the-counter medications) for both the brand name and the generic name or names. Sometimes you may find one but not the other on this list. If a prescribed drug is followed by +++ or ++++, read the relevant sections of this book to see whether the risk is great or small. Then confer with your physician to see how pressing the need for the drug truly is. Finally, take it if your or your baby's health depends upon it.

The ? and + are not endorsements. Remember, no drugs are known to be safe during pregnancy. These notations simply mean that the drug is not known to be harmful, or that it is probably less harmful than another ++, +++, or ++++ drug. But there is a big difference between "not known to be harmful" and "known to be safe." We discuss why in some detail in Chapter 8.

KNOWN OR SUSPECTED RISKS
OF VARIOUS DRUGS
TAKEN DURING PREGNANCY

Legend—

   ?   The drug has not been sufficiently well studied to date to allow useful or accurate recommendations. If possible avoid these, particularly during the first trimester.

   +   Some studies have been performed and no serious fetal consequences have yet been identified. This doesn't mean the drug is safe. It merely means that it *may be* relatively safe.

  ++   Some studies or theoretical considerations suggest *possible* hazards to the fetus or embryo.

++++   Some studies have *conclusively demonstrated hazards* to the fetus or embryo.

	First Trimester	Second Trimester	Third Trimester	Labor and Delivery
Acetaminophen	?	?	?	?
Adrenal cortex hormones	++	+	+	+
Alcohol (small)	+	+	+	+
Alcohol (large)	++++	++++	++++	++++
ALKA-SELTZER	+	+	+	++
ALLEREST	?	?	?	?
Aluminum Hydroxide	++	+	+	+
Aminophylline	?	?	?	?
Amphetamines	+++	++	++	++
ANACIN	++	++	++	++++
Aspirin	+	+	+	++
ARM	?	?	?	?
Barbiturates (small)	+	+	+	++
Barbiturates (large)	+	+	+	++
Belladonnas	+	+	+	+
BENDECTINE	+	+	+	+
Birth Control Pills	++	++	++	
BONINE	++	+	+	+
BUFFERIN	+++	++	++	++++
Caffeine	++	++	++	++
Cephaloridine	++	++	++	++
Cephalothin	++	++	++	++
Chloramphenicol	++	++	+++	++++
Chlorothiazide	++	++	++	++
Chlorpheniramine	?	?	?	?
Codeine (small)	+	+	+	++
Codeine (large)	+++	+++	++++	++++
COMPOZ	?	?	?	?
CONTAC	?	?	?	?
CORICIDIN	++	++	++	++++
Coumarin	+++	++	+++	++++
Cyclizine	++	+	+	++

	First Trimester	Second Trimester	Third Trimester	Labor and Delivery
Cyclopropane	++	+	+	+++
DARVON	+++	++	++	+++
DARVON COMPOUND	?	?	?	?
DATRIL	+	+	+	++++
Demerol (small)	+	+	+	++++
Demerol (large)	+++	+++	+++	?
Dextromethorphan	?	?	?	?
Diazepam	+++	++	++	+++
Diethylstilbestrol	++++			
DILANTIN	+++	+	+	+
Dimenhydrinate	+	+	+	+
Diphenhydramine	++	++	++	++
DOAN'S PILLS	++	++	++	+++
DRISTAN	++	++	++	++
EMPIRIN	?	?	?	?
Ephedrine	++	++	++	++
EQUANIL	+++	++	++	++
Erythromycin	+	+	+	+
Ethacrinic Acid	++	++	++	+++
EXCEDRIN	+++	++	++	++
EX-LAX	+	+	+	+
FLAGYL	++	+	+	+
Folic Acid	+	+	+	+
4-WAY COLD TABLETS	+++	++	++	++
Furosemide	++	+++	++	++
Gentamycin	++	++	++	++
GELUSIL	+	+	+	+
GERITOL	++	++	++	+++
Halothane	++	+	+	+++
Heparin	+	+	+	+
HEROIN (large)	+++	++	++++	+++
Hydralazine	+	+	++	++
Hydrochlorothiazide	++	++	++	+++
Hydroxyzine	++	+	+	+
Influenza Vaccine	+	+	+	+
Insulin	+	+	+	+
Iodides	+++	++	++	++
Isoproterenol	++	++	++	++
Kanamycin	+	+	+	+
Kaopectate	+	+	+	+
LIBRIUM	+++	++	++	++
LSD	++	++	++	++
MAALOX	+	+	+	+
Magnesium Hydroxide	+	+	+	+
MARAZINE	+	+	+	++
Marijuana	?	?	?	?
Meclizine	++	++	++	++
Meprobamate	+++	++	++	++
METHOTREXATE	++++			
Methyldopa	?	?	?	?
Methylphenidate	?	?	?	?
Metronidazole	+++	++	++	++
MILTOWN	+	+	+	+
Morphine (small)	+	+	+	++++
Morphine (large)	+++	+++	+++	+++
Nitrofurantoins	+	+	+	+
Nitrous Oxide	?	?	?	?
NYTOL	?	?	?	?
NY QUIL	?	?	?	?
Paregoric	+	+	+	++
Penicillin	?	?	?	?
Pentazocine	+	+	+	++
PERCODAN (small)	+++	++	++	++++
PERCODAN (large)	?	?	?	?
Phenacetin	?	?	?	?
Pheniramine	++	?	?	+++
Phenobarbital	+++	++	++	?
Phenteramine	?	?	++	

	First Trimester	Second Trimester	Third Trimester	Labor and Delivery
Phenylephrine	?	?	?	?
Phenylpropanolamine	?	?	?	?
PREPARATION H	+	+	+	+
Promethazine	++	++	++	+++
Propoxyphene	++	++	++	+++
Pyridoxine	+	+	+	+
Pyrilamine	?	?	?	?
Quinine	+++	+++	+++	+++
Reserpine	++	++	++	++++
ROBITUSSIN	?	?	?	++++
SINAREST	?	?	?	?
SINE OFF	+++	++	++	+++
SINE-AID	+++	++	++	++++
SINUTAB	?	?	?	?
SLEEP-EZE	?	?	?	?
SOMINEX	++	++	+	++
Sodium Bicarbonate	+	+	+	+
Sulfonamides	+	+	+	++
TALWIN	?	?	?	?
Tetracyclines	?	+++	+++	++
Theophylline	?	?	?	?
TIGAN	+++	+++	++	+++
Tolbutamide	++	++	++	++
Tricyclic Antidepressants	++	++	++	++
Trimethobenzamide	+	+	+	+
Tripelennamine	?	?	?	++
TYLENOL	?	?	?	?
Vitamin A*	+++	+++	++	++
Vitamin B's	+	+	+	+
Vitamin C	?	?	?	?
Vitamin D	+++	+++	++	++
Vitamin E	+	+	+	+
Vitamin K	+	+	+++	+
VALIUM	+++	+++	+++	++++
VANQUISH	+++	++	++	++++

Notes—

1. The notations ?, +, ++, +++, ++++ indicate that we know about the hazards, but they don't indicate how great the hazards actually are. In other words, all drugs with ++++ are *known* to present certain hazards to the unborn child. However, all drugs with ++++ are not equally hazardous. The extent of the risk is discussed in early chapters.
2. The notations "small" and "large" are used with a variety of addicting and abused drugs. "Small" refers to the usual dosage employed for valid medical indications. "Large" applies to excessive dosages characteristic of illict or addictive use.
3. * The dangers of vitamins refers to massive quantities occasionally used by food faddists. Usual recommended dosages given in Chapter 6, are generally believed to be both safe and necessary.

GLOSSARY

ANESTHETIC—A drug that is used to eliminate or reduce pain, generally for birth or surgery.

BIRTH DEFECT—Any abnormality, visible or not, which exists from the time of birth.

CONGENITAL—Referring to conditions that are present at birth.

DRUGS—Chemical compounds that are used to diagnose, prevent or treat diseases or other abnormal conditions.

EMBRYO—Name given to the infant in the uterus after differentiation begins and up to the point when all of the organs are formed (approximately weeks two to twelve).

FETUS—Name given to the infant in the uterus after the organs are fully formed until birth (approximately weeks twelve to forty).

INTRAUTERINE—Inside the mother's uterus (womb).

INTERVILLOUS SPACE—The part of the placenta which contains the mother's blood and which serves as one of the exchange areas between mother and child.

NARCOTIC—A class of drugs that relieves pain and impairs consciousness. Most are addicting. Includes heroin, morphine, Demerol, Percodan, codeine and others.

PLACENTA—The organ that attaches the mother to the growing child. It serves as an exchange site for oxygen, carbon dioxide, nutrients, wastes. It makes a variety of hormones and carries on many other functions that are essential to maintain the pregnancy.

RADIATION—A number of energy forms that travel through the air. Includes light wave and particulate forms. X rays are an example.

TERATOGENIC—Producing birth defects.

UMBILICAL CORD—The structure that carries blood from the baby to the placenta and back. It houses the umbilical artery and the umbilical veins through which the blood actually flows.

VILLUS—That part of the placenta which contains the tiny artery, capillary and vein that make up the final path of the fetal circulation. Here the fetal blood transfers and exchanges materials with the maternal blood in the intervillous spaces.

INDEX

237

ABOUT THE AUTHORS

RONALD E. GOTS, M.D., Ph.D., is the author of *The Truth about Medical Malpractice*. His PhD. is in pharmacology. BARBARA GOTS, M.D., M.A., is a graduate of the University of Southern California medical school. They have two young children.

THE FAMILY—TOGETHER AND APART

Choose from this potpourri of titles for the information you need on the many facets of family living.

Congratulations— But...

What about all those questions and problems that arrive with a new addition to the family? Here are several invaluable books for any new or expectant mother. They are filled with helpful hints for raising healthy children in a happy home. Best of luck and may all your problems be little ones!

Bantam Book Catalog

Here's your up-to-the-minute listing of over 1,400 titles by your favorite authors.

This illustrated, large format catalog gives a description of each title. For your convenience, it is divided into categories in fiction and non-fiction—gothics, science fiction, westerns, mysteries, cookbooks, mysticism and occult, biographies, history, family living, health, psychology, art.

So don't delay—take advantage of this special opportunity to increase your reading pleasure.

Just send us your name and address and 50¢ (to help defray postage and handling costs).

BANTAM BOOKS, INC.
Dept. FC, 414 East Golf Road, Des Plaines, Ill. 60016

Mr./Mrs./Miss_____
(please print)

Address_____

City_____State_____Zip_____

Do you know someone who enjoys books? Just give us their names and addresses and we'll send them a catalog too!

_____

Mr./Mrs./Miss_____

Address_____

City_____State_____Zip_____

_____

Mr./Mrs./Miss_____

Address_____

City_____State_____Zip_____

FC—9/78